Don't give me eggs that bounce

118 cracking recipes for people with Alzheimer's

*Peter Morgan-Jones, Emily Colombage,
Danielle McIntosh, Prudence Ellis*

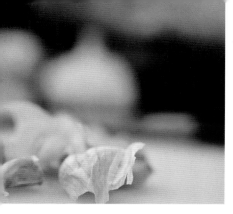
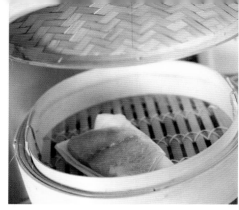
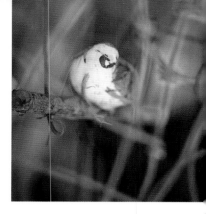
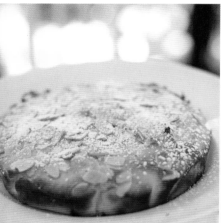
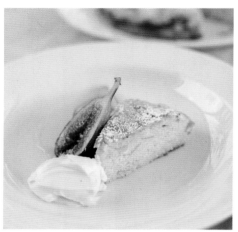
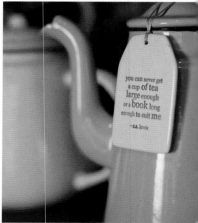
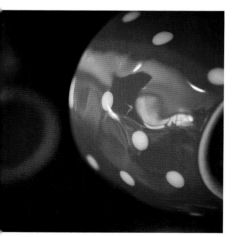
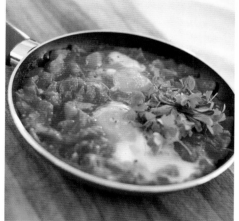
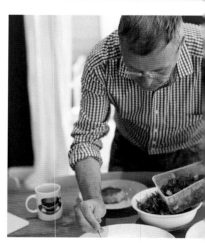
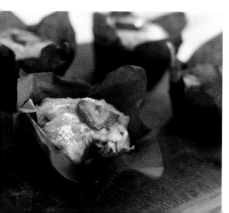
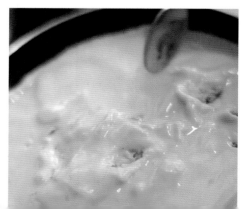
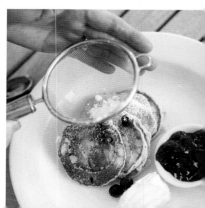

you can never get
a cup of tea
large enough
or a book long
enough to suit me
— c.s. lewis

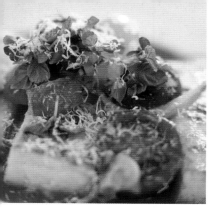
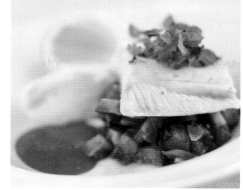
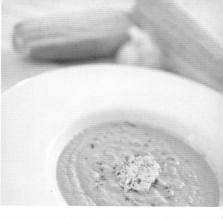
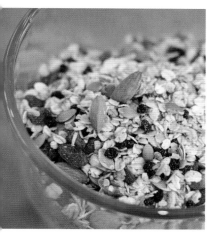
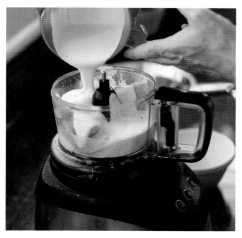
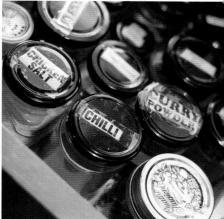
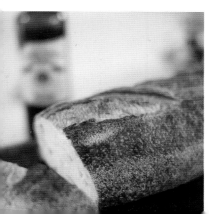
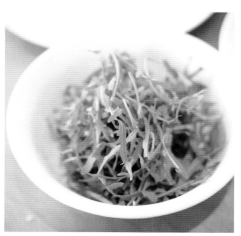
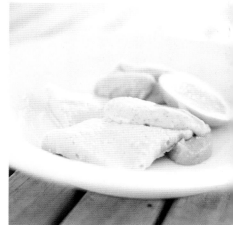
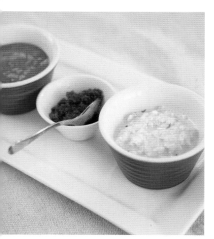
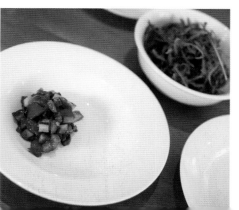
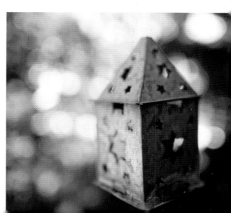

Contents

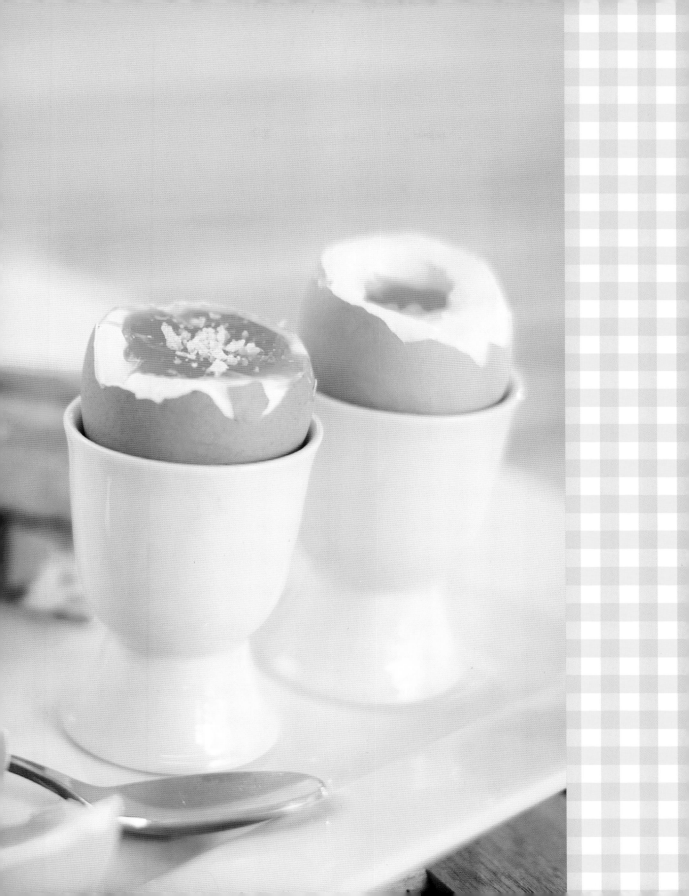

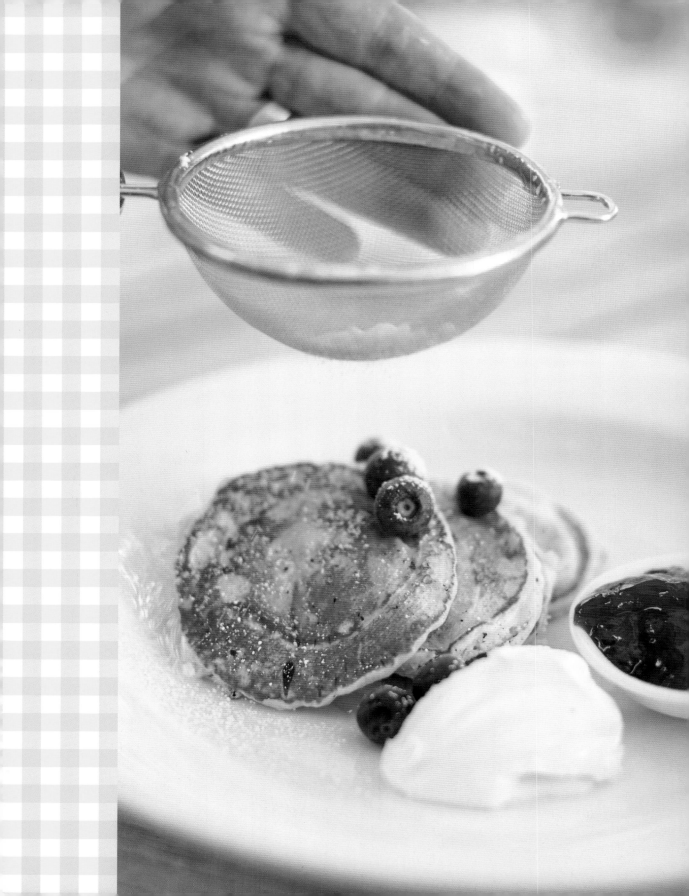

Foreword by Maggie Beer

I can't tell you how proud I am to be asked to write the foreword for this truly exciting, important book. Reading through I was blown away by the practical knowledge shared in such a readable way.

Don't give me eggs that bounce in fact gives people already in the field—so many of us who share a passion to see those in aged care or with dementia enjoy beautiful food—a wealth of ideas to make a difference for those we owe a duty of loving care to, whether people are in dementia care, aged care or at home with family carers.

I have to start by telling the story of how I came to know Peter Morgan-Jones, as he has been instrumental in changing many lives, mine included. When I was Senior Australian of the Year in 2010, among the 900 or so speaking requests I received, one came from the organisers of the annual conference of CEOs of aged care, held that year in Hobart. That was the first time I heard of Dr Stephen Judd of HammondCare and although we didn't actually meet at the conference we became aware of each other.

I had done a lot of research in the paper I was to give, such as visiting aged care homes and Meals on Wheels to understand some of the problems and complexities, to form my ideas for the paper. Wanting to go with possible solutions, I bothered my friends in the industry for ideas on delicious food to be made for large numbers that were cost effective and full of flavour as a discussion point of what was possible.

I could never say the talk was an unqualified success as I felt a particular chill in the air as I talked, giving examples of the great—but also the terrible things—I had encountered.

I talked of the need to change the culture of food in aged care and to give all residents a beautiful meal every day to look forward to. And all of the things that would need to change for that to happen for all.

It was the most difficult talk I ever gave but out of it came some enormous good. The most visible sign of that was the meeting in Sydney with Dr Judd to talk about the best way to provide a catalyst for change. I've always said that change can't happen without great leadership and this was certainly so here and the result of the ideas around the table that day was the choosing of Peter Morgan-Jones to be the Executive Chef and Food Ambassador—to be that catalyst for change for HammondCare and beyond.

Having followed Peter's work, I have basked in the knowledge that he has acquired and I've seen the change he has been able to make. The excitement he brings to his task; his passion for food and people and the change it can make for those living with dementia not only spurred him on, so ably supported by HammondCare staff such as Dietitian Emily Colombage, but many of us around Australia who are so concerned for those who are in facilities where food is offered without any joy or love.

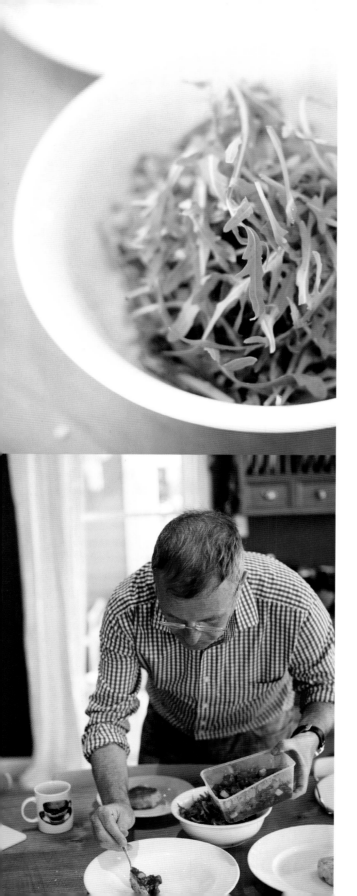

'The knowledge in these pages will help so many of us drive change to give those in need the joy of beautiful food and all that comes with it.'

That day in Hobart, the meeting with Dr Judd and following Peter's work, has led me to continue on that journey I started back in 2010 but with far more knowledge than I began with. The knowledge in these pages will help so many of us drive change to give those in need the joy of beautiful food and all that comes with it.

There is no doubt, changing a culture is an incredibly complex issue. To read the chapter by Prudence Ellis, Speech Pathologist of Braeside Hospital, about people with swallowing difficulties or Danielle McIntosh, Senior Dementia Consultant of the Dementia Centre, and her chapter on positive mealtimes for people with dementia, shows that there is so much more than food that has to be taken into account, but what a wonderful beginning this book gives us all.

The more knowledge we can share the more we can combat the problems that do exist so that every person—no matter their age or infirmity—has the chance of beautiful, nutritious food in their day. It should be everyone's right and this book will be so important in that journey.

Maggie Beer

Introduction

Eggs as they should be

Eggs cooked just the way you like them are one of the great symbols of choice, health and flavour in food. But when it comes to food for older people and those with dementia, too often eggs have come to symbolise just the opposite.

When HammondCare's Chief Executive, Dr Stephen Judd, wrote about eggs served to some older people as being more like 'kiln-fired organic pottery' than real eggs, he sparked a conversation that has led all the way to this book, and beyond.

This passion to ensure great food for older people and people living with dementia inspired the appointment of Peter Morgan-Jones as HammondCare's Executive Chef and Food Ambassador.

And, as Maggie Beer says in her foreword, these steps also impacted her own campaign to see 'that every person—no matter the age or the infirmity—has the chance of beautiful, nutritious food in their day'.

Don't give me eggs that bounce: 118 cracking recipes for people with Alzheimer's is a deliberately provocative title aimed at continuing this important food conversation.

And the book takes it further—directly empowering carers, people living with dementia and other vulnerable people by providing 'cracking' original recipes and extensive practical knowledge about how to make food and dining a positive and memorable experience.

We know carers already work tirelessly to provide this for their loved ones and we are confident that *Don't give me eggs that bounce* will provide much-needed support. We also hope this book will influence the delivery of food globally in dementia and aged care so that, in the words of Peter Morgan-Jones, he will receive no further reports of older people being served 'eggs like ping-pong balls'.

Don't give me eggs that bounce celebrates— and hopes to give voice to—the dignity of older people, people with dementia and those with eating disabilities by offering innovative, nutritious, glorious food, where the 'flavours do the talking'. All in the context of being carefully analysed and clinically appropriate. No compromise on taste, no compromise on safety.

As 'cracking' as Peter's recipes are, they are not the only feature of this book. He has also shared his innovations about preparing and presenting modified foods, which have been so well received in HammondCare's dementia cottages. His work is vitally supported by expert chapters on nutrition, diet, swallowing and eating issues, texture-modified foods and successful dining with dementia from co-authors Emily Colombage, Danielle McIntosh and Prudence Ellis—see 'About the authors'.

People, like a good meal, have unique ingredients

Everyone is unique. Our life experiences, personality and relationships all impact how we see the world, how we react, what we enjoy and even how a person lives with dementia and other conditions.

What might work well for some may not assist everyone. This is especially true for one of the most personal of human experiences, the enjoyment of food. The best-practice strategies in this book may not all work for every reader. However we are confident that at least some of our strategies, food tips and recipes will make a lasting difference in your life and family.

Not only dementia

Don't give me eggs that bounce has been written specifically for people living with Alzheimer's and dementia, however the recipes and strategies may also help people living with other conditions. Our ideas that help with good nutrition, swallowing and environmental support may benefit people with a range of health issues or disabilities. It's our hope that *Don't give me eggs that bounce* will help ensure more people—regardless of their age or health—are supported to enjoy great eating and drinking experiences.

To set the scene for *Don't give me eggs that bounce*, let's consider what Alzheimer's and dementia are and how they can impact on a person's experience of eating and drinking.

A few words about dementia

Different types of dementia

Alzheimer's Disease International (2011)[1] estimates that there are about 36 million people worldwide living with dementia, and by 2030, this will rise to 66 million.

The term dementia is used to describe a range of progressive disorders that affect the brain. It is mainly a condition of older age. The person with dementia can experience a number of symptoms including:

- impaired memory
- disorientation
- poor concentration
- difficulty in naming and use of language
- impaired ability to learn, or recall learnt information
- difficulty with motor skills and coordination
- difficulty with thinking and in understanding or following a sequence.

The significant cognitive impairments caused by dementia can be accompanied by personality and mood changes in the individual and changes in their judgement.

Dementia is principally an umbrella term used to describe a number of conditions in which these symptoms occur. Alzheimer's disease, the most common type of dementia, is characterised by a gradual but persistent decline in cognitive functioning.

Vascular or multi-infarct dementia, is characterised by a step-wise decline where the person has a series of vascular accidents or problems with circulation to the brain that destroy areas of the brain. Dementia with Lewy bodies is characterised by fluctuations in cognitive impairment, hallucinations and falls.

There are other conditions that, as they progress, may also result in dementia. These include Parkinson's disease, Huntington's disease, infections (such as HIV and Creutzfeldt-Jakob disease) and excessive alcohol use.

For more information about dementia, speak to your doctor, specialist, or Alzheimer's advisory organisation.

Supporting independence

Whatever the cause of dementia, the path of the disease does lead to a loss of independence. While dementia cannot be cured, we can support the person living with dementia to keep their sense of independence, dignity and control—as much and for as long as possible—by putting into practice good support strategies.

These strategies, including those for food, are influenced by knowing that a person with a diagnosis of dementia may feel vulnerable and frightened and need reassurance and support. But also that they—depending on the progression of the disease—hold views and opinions, have a strong sense of identity, want to do things for themselves and understand what is happening to them in the early stages.

Dementia, eating and drinking?

Most of us don't think a great deal about the daily process of eating and drinking. We take it for granted that we can decide what we feel like and how best to fulfil desires for food or drink. But imagine if your efforts to meet these basic needs were constantly thwarted or interfered with? Dementia can have that impact, which is why this book is so important.

Don't give me eggs that bounce discusses the most common food-related challenges for people with dementia and carers and provides advice, strategies and suggestions.

Whether it is losing weight and nutritional deficiencies; difficulty chewing, swallowing or using cutlery; or challenges of attention span and communicating choices, our strategies developed from research and experience focus on learning to understand these difficulties and how to provide support.

Don't give me eggs that bounce is a useful first step, one we hope will become a regular part of your food life, but please know that you are not on your own in this journey. The 'Contact and resources' section provides details of organisations and support services that can help.

As mentioned, the authors of this book have extensive experience caring for people with dementia, both in residential care and at home. But if some of the strategies and recipes here do not work for you, perhaps you may be inspired to adjust or improve on them so that they do.

We would love to hear readers' tips and suggestions so that we can share them with others. See 'Contacts and resources' or visit crackingrecipes.com

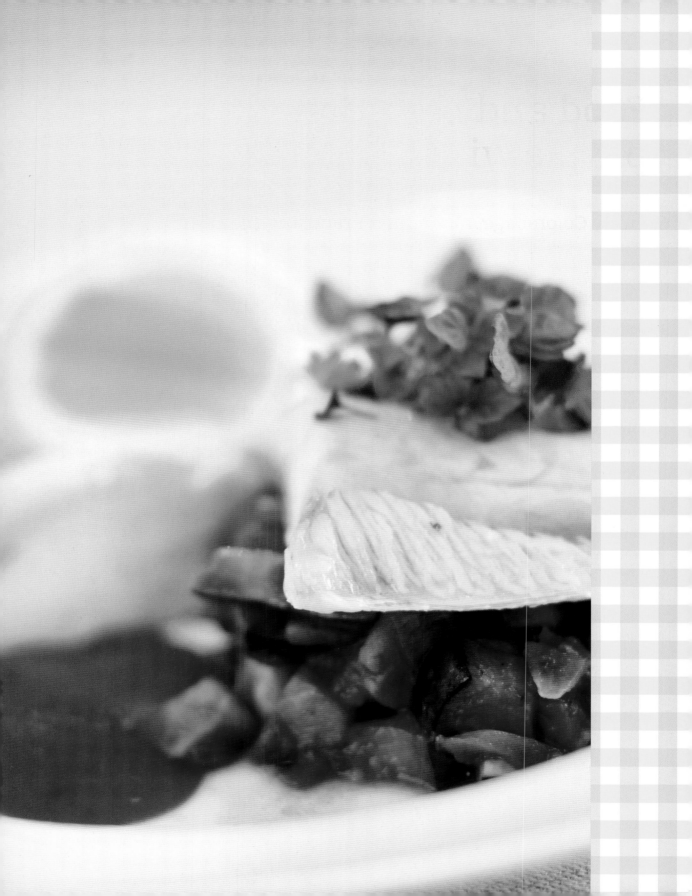

Food and nutrition for people with dementia

Emily Colombage, Accredited Practising Dietitian

Food is vital for people living with Alzheimer's and other dementias, both for enjoyment and good nutrition. That's why *Don't give me eggs that bounce* presents food that is appetising, tasty and nutritious with a special focus on energy and protein rather than low fat, salt or sugar.

When someone is living with a degenerative illness such as dementia, the usual nutrition and health messages often no longer apply. It is important to get good medical advice before imposing any dietary limitations, including those that have been recommended in the past. This is especially the case if someone is struggling with weight loss or a poor appetite.[2]

What's malnutrition got to do with it?

When we hear the word malnutrition our minds usually picture an underweight child in a developing country. Many people are surprised to learn that malnutrition occurs all around us in older people and people living with certain diseases. Often people living with dementia experience malnutrition (or under-nutrition) and about 10 to 30 per cent[3] of people receiving community care are malnourished.

Dementia, as well as the effects of ageing, can cause minimal appetite, loss of smell and taste, disinterest in food, confusion at mealtime and difficulty with chewing and swallowing. Some people living with dementia also experience short attention spans or agitation, which increases their energy output—meaning they need to eat more to compensate. People living in the community may have additional challenges in accessing food and being able to prepare it. See Chapter 6 for suggestions for carers.

There are unhealthy consequences when the body does not receive enough energy (calories or kilojoules) and protein. Weight loss causes the body to lose fat and accelerates the decrease in muscle mass that already occurs as we age. Weight loss causes lethargy and increased frailty while reduced muscle mass results in loss of strength and physical ability to do everyday tasks. Weight loss also increases the likelihood of falling, weakens skin integrity and the ability to fight infections. It can also reduce cognition and affect overall enjoyment of life.

Some people might be eating and/or drinking poorly due to treatable factors such as reflux, constipation, swallowing difficulties, painful teeth or depression. If a person with dementia is losing weight unintentionally you should always see your doctor to improve any of these treatable concerns.

Strategies for good nutrition

A range of strategies can assist a person living with dementia to have good nutrition. Some may be ongoing, while others may only be useful short-term. As dementia progresses, the time may come to replace one strategy with another.

The main strategies that people find helpful include:

- high energy and protein foods
- finger foods
- eating more often
- creative solutions at the dinner table
- supplements
- environment and dining (Chapter 2)
- texture-modified foods and fluids (Chapter 3).

High energy and protein foods

When someone is undernourished and living with dementia, they need foods high in nutrition that prioritise calories and protein. People with dementia may only eat small amounts because their appetite is reduced or because eating takes so much effort.

Our aim should be to make the most of every mouthful and not waste stomach space or effort with foods that are low in nutrients.

A good approach is to choose foods that are naturally high in energy and protein such as custard and cheese, or enriching a regular food to increase the nutrients. For example, adding some cream or cheese when making a vegetable soup.

To increase calorie intake, full cream dairy products and full fat products should be used. 'Diet' or 'low calorie' products should be avoided. Also, it is extremely important to consume enough protein. Rich sources of protein include eggs, meat, fish and dairy foods.

Fabulous finger foods

The experience of being fed can be invasive and disempowering. Finger foods can help people maintain independence and dignity at mealtimes if the person is having physical difficulty eating or concentrating on food. They give people greater control of what goes into their mouth. Finger foods aim to enable independence and remove some of the frustration that mealtimes can bring.

Importantly, finger foods are much more than frozen party pies and mini-quiches, as our recipes show. Finger foods can be high in energy and protein or part of a normal, healthy, balanced diet. Examples of finger food include:

- thickly sliced meats
- cheese blocks
- boiled eggs
- steamed broccoli
- cauliflower florets
- halved cherry tomatoes
- finger sandwiches.

Many of our recipes are suitable for finger foods and are high in energy and protein. See my finger food ideas table at the end of this chapter and finger foods in our 'Meal plans' section. If a person is recommended a modified diet, check with your speech pathologist as to which finger food options are compliant.

Eating more often

With short attention spans and reduced appetites, small and frequent meals can be a helpful response. Eating five to seven small meals can result in a greater overall intake across the day compared to three big meals. People with a poor appetite can find the sight of a big plate of food overwhelming and even sickening.

Food presentation is very important in tempting someone to eat. Try presenting smaller portions and if they are still hungry they can come back for seconds.

Morning teas, afternoon teas and supper can serve an important role in this approach. As well as the recipes presented in this book, other quick and easy, high energy and high protein mini-meals include:

- milkshakes or smoothies
- flavoured milk
- creamy (full fat) yoghurt
- individual dairy desserts (fridge section of supermarket)
- milo, hot chocolate or Ovaltine with full cream milk
- instant coffee made with milk, cappuccino, latte
- creamed rice in a can
- cream cheese spread and crackers
- pre-made custard cups (shelf stable or in refrigerated section of the supermarket)
- ricotta or cream cheese with honey on toast or biscuit
- savoury dips or cream cheese with vegetable sticks or crackers
- sardines, kippers or herring fillets on toast
- raisin toast or croissants with lots of butter
- peanut butter or cheese sandwiches
- premade rissoles, falafels or arancini balls
- olives, salami, cabanossi, cheese
- shortbread or meringue
- scones or pikelets
- fruit or carrot cake with margarine or icing.

Creative solutions at the dinner table

Carers and people living with dementia may often find mealtimes stressful.

Dementia can change what a person likes to eat. This can be a frustrating experience for carers who work hard preparing a favourite meal only to find their loved one no longer enjoys that food. This may be because it has become too difficult to chew or swallow, or taste changes. Also, a particular diet may be recommended for health reasons, but the reasoning behind this is not well understood by the person with dementia.

In dealing with these changes it might be helpful to ask:

- Is it really important that a particular food or drink is consumed?
- If yes, or if the person is eating very little, can you get creative with solutions, with the help of your local doctor or a dietitian?

A person's food preferences may simply change and it is usually best to just accept this. Get creative and experiment. For example, instead of agonising over another wasted steak (which used to be a favourite), try more tender red meat cooked in a casserole or using mince.

If using cutlery is the problem, try using finger foods like sliced roast meat or meatballs. If the person you cook for is becoming disinterested in savoury foods and losing weight, why not offer more sweet foods? Anecdotally, many carers report people living with dementia grow to prefer sweet foods. Fortunately there are lots of sweet foods high in energy and protein (these are primarily dairy based foods, such as milkshakes, ice cream or custard).

Older people are also at risk of not having enough fluids, fibre, vitamin B12, calcium, vitamin D and iron. If creative solutions are not enough, sometimes a multivitamin or a fibre supplement (Metamucil or Benefibre) might be the best option. It is recommended you consult your doctor or dietitian before starting any of these.

Fluids are also very important and a person should aim to have eight glasses of fluid a day. Some options to boost fluid intake include using ice blocks, jelly, ice creams, soft drink or custard as these still contain high fluid levels. If a person is recommended thickened drinks, check with your speech pathologist to ensure these are compliant and do not risk the safety of the person.

People on texture-modified diets, particularly minced and moist and smooth pureed, can be at risk of not consuming enough carbohydrate. This can happen when the usual sources of carbohydrates are not allowed or are difficult to prepare (for example: sandwiches, toast, breakfast cereals, rice and pasta). It is important to ensure carbohydrates are still included in the diet. Look for our recipe ideas involving potato, semolina and ground rice.

What about supplements?

Supplements—special high energy and protein drinks—are another tool to reduce weight loss and malnutrition. The wide range of supplements on the market include powders mixed with milk or water and pre-made drinks. Some have higher calories or are juice flavoured, while some are pre-thickened for people who required thickened fluids. A number of the powdered supplements are available cheaply at discount pharmacies. Others are available at normal pharmacies but at a higher cost.

The cheapest supplement is milk powder (add ¼ cup of full cream milk powder to a cup of full cream milk and mix well).

The role of a dietitian

Dietitians are experts in food and nutrition and will conduct a nutritional assessment to develop a nutrition care plan and support you in its implementation. They can also assist with practical strategies to help clients improve nutrition.

Dietitians are able to decide whether supplements are necessary and, if they are, can organise for them to be delivered at reduced cost. People holding Department of Veteran's Affairs gold cards are also able to purchase supplements at reduced cost.

For details on how to find a dietitian near you, see 'Contacts and resources'.

Vegetables

Vegetables can be raw or cooked in different ways. Chopping into chunks before cooking makes them easier to pick up and look nicer. Some people will manage better with softer veggies. Options include:

- cooked broccoli or cauliflower florets
- roast potato, sweet potato or pumpkin
- small boiled potatoes
- potato chips, wedges or potato cakes
- Brussels sprouts or button mushrooms cooked and halved
- steamed green beans, asparagus or snow peas
- cucumber or capsicum chunks
- mini or finger eggplants, cooked
- halved cherry tomatoes or regular tomatoes in wedges
- steamed zucchini or carrot chunks
- cucumber or capsicum chunks
- corn fritters
- lentil, chickpea or vegetable patties/rissoles
- vegetable soup in a mug
- gnocchi.

Meat, poultry, fish and alternatives

Meat needs to be very tender. Cutting meat into bite sized pieces before the cooking process can improve presentation. Options include:

- chicken breast or thigh, cut into bite-sized pieces
- hamburgers, meatballs, rissoles, (try beef, lamb, chicken or pork for variety)
- roast tender meat sliced
- lamb cutlets
- sausages or chipolatas cooked and sliced in chunks
- ham slices or salami sticks
- pieces of fish (boned), fish fingers, herring or kippers
- slices of quiche or frittata cut into squares
- hard-boiled eggs (quartered)
- thin omelette rolled and sliced
- tofu squares
- lentil, chickpea patties/rissoles.

Breads and cereals

Plenty of variety here and don't forget to add butter or margarine
- toast or bread fingers
- mini bread rolls, panini or naan
- popcorn
- rice cakes
- raisin toast or fruit cake
- pita bread cut into smaller pieces
- crumpets
- English muffins or scones
- soft cereal bars
- crispbread
- penne, ravioli or other bigger pasta shapes
- Nutrigrain.

Fruit

Some fruity suggestions include:
- apple, banana, kiwi fruit or pear wedges or chunks
- tropical fruit in slices such as melons, pineapple
- citrus segments such as mandarin, orange or grapefruit
- whole strawberries, raspberries or mulberries
- peach or nectarine in wedges (leaving skin on can provide grip)
- halved and deseeded plum or apricot
- dried fruit such as apricot halves, prunes or dates
- seedless grapes.

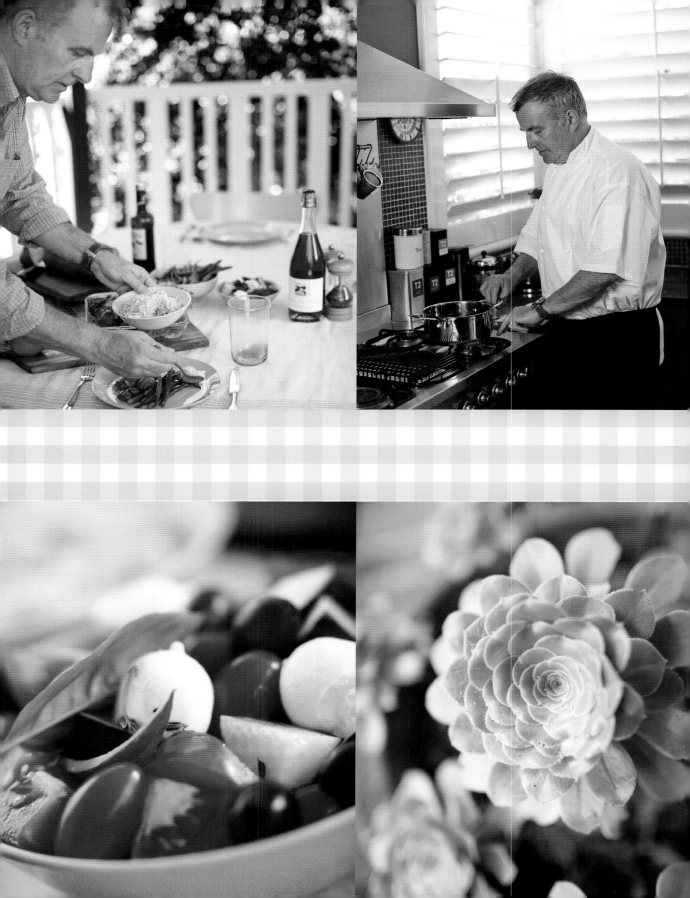

Positive dining and successful eating

Danielle McIntosh, Senior Dementia Consultant

A better understanding of how to support a person to eat and drink can make a positive difference to their health, self-esteem and quality of life.

Common eating and drinking difficulties for a person with dementia may include not recognising food and cutlery, not being able to perform eating/drinking steps in the right order, as well as changed behaviours.

It is not just dementia that can create difficulties with eating and drinking—age related changes also play a major role. When people age, there are sensory impairments (failing eyesight, cataracts, glaucoma and poor hearing) as well as physical changes and conditions (arthritis in joints especially fingers, decaying teeth or using dentures, lower energy levels) which impact how a person functions. These can also affect their emotional state, as eating and drinking for many people is central to how they view quality of life.

Eating and drinking difficulties can reduce the enjoyment of some of our favourite activities as they may:

- take longer

- require more energy

- make a person feel different/disabled/hopeless

- require different food/drink textures, crockery and cutlery

- isolate someone from friends and family.

In response, a range of strategies will be helpful in supporting the person with dementia to eat and drink as independently as possible while addressing the most common issues.

'Eating and drinking difficulties can reduce the enjoyment of some of our favourite activities.'

Words	Body Language
Use simple words and phrases	Appear calm
Speak with a clear voice and at the speed that the person can understand (ensure you allow them enough time to respond)	Don't look rushed—take your time
Use words that are appropriate and familiar to the person	Show that you want to eat and drink with the person
Be positive (avoid sarcasm, condescending and childish words and tones)	Display interest in the person by maintaining eye contact, talking and sitting with them to eat
Offer a person choice (but limit it to two to three things as too much choice may be confusing)	Smile—this helps people relax, both those who receive it and who give it!
	Gain the person's attention
	Give the person your attention by maintaining eye contact, listening and observing their body language

'A person with dementia may be distracted by noise and movement in the environment...'

Know the person

It may seem obvious, but reflecting on the meals and types of food and drink that are—and have been in the past—important to the person can help make eating and drinking a successful experience. Things like:

- What food/drink does a person like or dislike?

- What food/drink holds good or bad memories?

- When does the person like to eat/drink?

  > Is breakfast when the person first wakes up or is it after they have a shower and get dressed?

  > Do they have a glass of water with lunch followed by a cup of tea?

  > Do they enjoy a piece of cheese and a drink of water during the night?

- What mealtime routines did the person follow (or perhaps have as a child)?

  > Washing face and hands before coming to the dining table.

  > Eating everything on their plate to avoid getting into trouble.

  > Setting the table and clearing their plate when finished.

- What food and drinks were special or gave particular comfort?

- Where did they usually—or especially like—to eat their meals?

  > For example, at the dining room table, in front of the television, having a morning cup of tea outside in the shaded backyard.

- How do they prefer food, drink or meals to be presented?

  > For example, using a specific plate/cup/mug, using napkins/serviettes, serving meals with a drink.

Try to keep the same routines and preferences for the person, as this helps them make sense of what they are seeing and keeps a sense of familiarity.

Think about physical environment

The physical layout and features of the space where a person eats and drinks can have a big impact on how well they function. This includes the room they are in, the table layout, the seating and how the food is positioned in relation to where they sit. Familiarity of the dining space is an important factor and there are several others.

Aiding concentration

A person with dementia may be distracted by noise and movement in the environment or may have difficulty with the correct sequence for eating/drinking. This can cause frustration, an unwillingness to eat and drink or result in the meal not being completed. Useful strategies include:

- Keeping the dining space quiet to help the person focus on eating—turn off the television or radio as this may compete for the person's attention.

- Avoiding use of mobile phones during mealtime.

- Not rushing—allowing plenty of time.

- Serving a combination of foods that can be eaten either sitting at the table or walking around, such as finger foods.

- Encouraging the person to eat and finish their meal, while not pressuring them. Some additional tips:

  > sit and eat with the person who may benefit from watching the steps and movements you make to eat.

  > limit (if possible) the number of people sitting at the table, especially if the person feels awkward or embarrassed eating in front of others.

  > if having a family meal, pay attention to seating arrangements such as positioning the person with dementia at the end of the table to help minimise distraction and next to people who understand the person's needs and can help them

  > seat people who eat quickly further away, as they may encourage the person with dementia to eat too quickly or to stop eating when the other person has finished.

  > seat people who tend to leave food on their plate further away, as this may signal to the person with dementia to stop eating or may encourage them to eat the food off the other person's plate.

Seeing clearly

Mashed potato, served on a white plate and placed on a white tablecloth can be hard to see for a person with poor eyesight. You can help recognition of food by using contrasting colours to highlight what you want them to see and positioning the meal and/or drink in the most visible way. Try:

- Contrasting plate colour with tablecloth colour.

- Using different coloured plates that don't blend in with the food.

- A white cup with a red or green coloured cordial drink.

- Placing the plate directly in front of the person and position the cup where the person is used to it being.

- Put out only the necessary cutlery for successfully eating the meal. Too many choices could be overwhelming.

- Make sure lighting in the room is good. Open curtains to let in natural light, turn on additional lights/lamps and change globes to higher wattages. Older people need two to three times as much light as younger people.

- Check the things sometimes overlooked—does the person have on their glasses? Are the glasses clean? When was the last time the prescription was reviewed?

Comfortable, supportive chair

Sitting in a chair that is comfortable and supportive is essential for a person with dementia. If they are uncomfortable, they may be restless or be unwilling to sit and this could result in not eating, having only small amounts or becoming upset when they are unable to communicate the problem. Make sure that:

- The chair is the right size—not too tight or too big for their body shape.

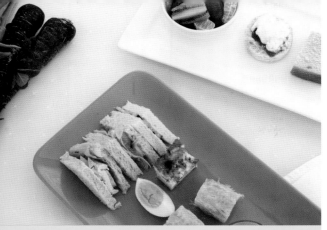

The white plate is less clear against the white tablecloth.

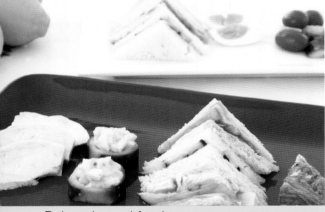

Pale coloured foods are more visible on a darker coloured plate.

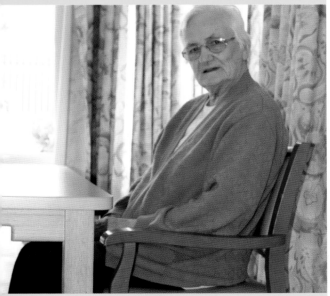

Sitting upright helps with safe swallowing.

- Their feet reach the floor—a foot stool is useful if the chair is too high.

- Their body is in good alignment with back and legs at a 90° angle.

- The table is not too high or low.

The general comfort of the chair is important. A chair with arms may feel more secure, especially if someone is tired during a meal or leans to the side. The seat of the chair needs to be comfortable enough for someone to sit for the length of a meal—a cushion on a hard seat can help. On the other hand, a cushioned seat may be too soft or worn out so a replacement should be considered. The back of the chair needs to offer good support. Cushions or rolls for supporting a person's back may be useful.

Knowing needs and challenges

Problems with cutlery

A person with dementia may not remember how to use cutlery. For many families and friends this can be distressing, in turn increasing a sense of hopelessness and dependence. Some useful strategies to try are:

- Offering a reminder to the person to use their 'spoon', 'fork', 'knife'.

- Only placing the necessary cutlery on the table.

- Sitting opposite the person and using your cutlery—this shows a person what to do which might be all the help they need.

- Placing the cutlery in the person's hand.

- Cutting up the person's food so that they only need to use a fork or spoon.

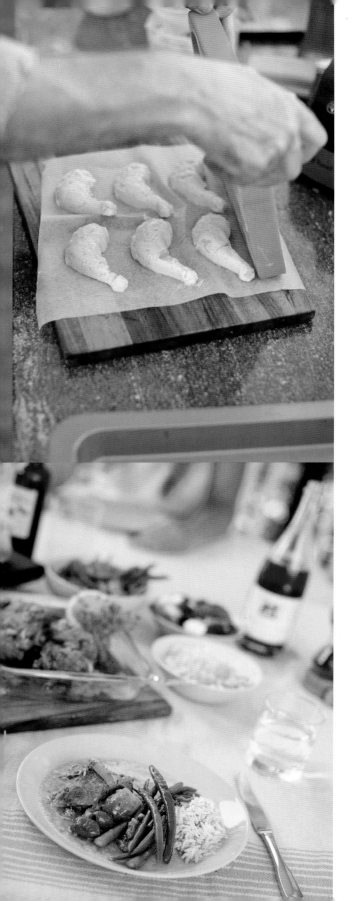

- Using cutlery the person is familiar with—if they have begun using adaptive cutlery, such as built up handles or angled spoons, this may cause additional confusion, so consider discontinuing their use.

- Accepting that cutlery can't be used anymore and preparing foods that can be eaten without it, such as finger foods (see our 'Recipes' section and also Chapter 1).

Not recognising food or mealtimes

A person with dementia sometimes may not know what to do when a meal or drink is placed in front of them. If they require texture-modified food or fluids, presentation is important to help the person know what they are eating–remember, you eat with your eyes as well as your mouth! Try:

- Using moulds to help a texture-modified meal look appetising and recognisable—see Chapter 5.

- Sitting and sharing a meal—it will encourage the person with dementia to eat as well.

- Explaining what the meal is.

- Keeping the meal simple—serve one course at a time and minimise garnishes.

- Helping a person know that it is mealtime through the normal sounds and smells of cooking food which are eating cues for us all. For example—toasting bread, making coffee, frying onions or garlic—these provide smells throughout the house that stimulate appetite.

- Encouraging the person with dementia to help with preparing or cooking the meal.

- Encouraging their assistance with pre-meal routines that they would normally perform or see, such as setting the table, washing hands, buttering bread.

- Giving gentle reminders may help a person know that it is time to eat. Where possible, use words or phrases that the person uses themselves or have been meaningful in the past. For example, 'dinner is ready', or 'time for a cuppa'.

Lack of appetite

Reduction in appetite is a common issue as people age and more specifically for people with dementia.

The strategies presented in Chapter 2 and many of the ideas already discussed in this chapter may assist to boost appetite. But there's more that can be done.

Making the meal a social event by inviting a small, select group of friends and family is a great aid to appetite. Eating the meal outside, especially in the person's favourite place is another great idea. This could be a garden, back verandah or even in the park.

Not too many people can resist the smell of a barbecue and encouraging the person with dementia to help with cooking may be an added boost to appetite. And if they really don't feel hungry, they may feel happy to have a drink instead.

Provide food and drink when the person indicates they are hungry. This includes in the middle of the night. Waking up hungry can impact on a person's ability to go back to sleep. A warm drink and a snack (such as honey on toast, slice of cheese or custard) could be beneficial.

Finally, for a busy carer or family member, keeping a diary of what their loved one eats and drinks each day may be useful when speaking with their doctor, dietitian, speech pathologist or other health professional.

Over-eating and not recognising when to stop

A person with dementia may start to over-eat, seek food constantly during the day or ask for second, third and fourth helpings. This can be because they:

- Have forgotten they have already eaten.

- Are not paying attention to or recognising the sensation of being 'full' because of damage to the brain.

- May crave certain foods—most commonly sweet foods.

- Are unsure of where they are and what is happening, so take as much food as they can or store it in a safe place.

In addressing overeating, develop or maintain the person's mealtime routines, including snacks throughout the day. Also, pace mealtime, providing space between courses and helpings. Pay attention to portion sizes by trying to serve small portions, but offering seconds if asked for more.

Availability of food is a factor—provide low calorie foods and snacks (such as fruit) on the kitchen bench or sideboard or where the person would normally have a fruit bowl so they can help themselves and feel secure that food is always available. Also, portion foods and place them in the cupboard or fridge. For example, rather than have a biscuit barrel filled to the top, have two biscuits in there at a time.

Some overeating may not be a negative thing if the person is enjoying their food, maintaining a healthy weight or needing to gain some weight. Exercise caution when considering if a person with dementia should lose weight as they will also lose muscle mass and this will have negative health consequences in the long term. Seek advice from your doctor or dietitian.

Feeling isolated and alone

A person with dementia is at greater risk of social isolation because of their needs and difficulties. Sometimes when friends and family do not know what is happening or how to help in relation to food, they feel awkward and will distance themselves.

Share this book, invite them for a meal and help them learn how to communicate with the person with dementia so that relationships can be maintained. Other strategies to try include:

- Have everyone eat the same meal (even if it is a texture-modified meal).

- Know the person with dementia and what they are able to do and what they need help with. This could include seating them next to someone who is confident to assist.

- Learn how long a person can tolerate noise and social interaction.

- Don't be afraid to go out to restaurants or other people's houses. However, preparation is the key. Make sure you know:

  > where the toilets are, and if you need to be close to them, discreetly request this from restaurant staff

  > know the best times to go to the restaurant, preferably avoiding busy periods

  > ask the restaurant to prepare and present meals/drinks a certain way or bring your own. Most restaurants are very willing to help you enjoy your meal and will do everything they can to provide support.

Eating or drinking the wrong things

When a person with dementia is hungry or thirsty they may choose something to eat or drink that is inappropriate or even dangerous. There are two vital principles for keeping your loved-one safe.

Keep inappropriate food/drink secure

Installing a lock on one or two cupboards in the kitchen and laundry allows chemicals to be stored safely. Keeping the locks and the cupboard doors discreet can be even better. For example, magnetic locks can be invisible.

Where possible avoid using padlocks or chains as this actually highlights the cupboard and signals that there is something 'forbidden' in there—humans are curious creatures and we like looking for hidden treasure!

Another idea is to change the look of one or two cupboard doors or drawers. Removing the handle from a door or cupboard can make them less obvious, or painting the cupboard door the same colour as the wall to disguise it may also help. In HammondCare's dementia homes these are known colloquially as 'Harry Potter doors'!

Make appropriate foods/fluids readily available

As well as making unsafe substances less obvious, it's vital that food and drink is easy to find. Do this by placing them in obvious places such as the kitchen bench, dining room table or sideboard.

If food or drink is in an over-bench cupboard, remove the door so that any food or cups placed there can be easily seen. Alternatively, replace the solid cupboard door with one that has a Perspex window to ensure the person with dementia can clearly see what is in the cupboard.

Finally, a label with the person's name on food and drink in the fridge or on the bench can reduce confusion or uncertainty.

Needing help to eat and drink

There are many types of modified cutlery, plates and cups that can help a person continue to feed themselves. For more information on modified equipment that could be useful or where to buy it, contact your local hospital's occupational therapy department or your state's Independent Living Centre ('Contacts and resources'). If you know what you need, many local chemists now stock some useful aids.

As dementia progresses, a person may find they need physical assistance to eat and drink. This should only be done when all other options for supporting a person have been tried because being physically assisted to eat and drink can be upsetting, frustrating and embarrassing.

It is important to be supportive and positive and many of the tips above and in other chapters may assist. In addition:

- Don't be anxious if it takes a person with dementia up to 45 minutes to eat their meal.
- Maintain the person's dignity at all times. This can include placing a napkin on their lap, rather than using a clothes protector or 'bib'.
- Sit down next to the person, so that you are at the same level.
- Gently touching the person's hand or arm can help them pay attention to you and eating/drinking.
- Speaking short words or phrases such as 'open your mouth', 'swallow' or 'chew' can help the person know what to do.
- Making sure that food and drink is served at the right temperature.
- Follow any instructions a speech pathologist or occupational therapist has recommended to support the person to eat and drink safely.
- For more information on how to help a person with swallowing difficulties—see Chapter 3.

If you know other strategies that work, we would love to hear about them. Sharing positive stories and strategies helps other carers and people with dementia enhance their enjoyment of eating and drinking, so please get in touch with The Dementia Centre—see 'Contacts and resources'.

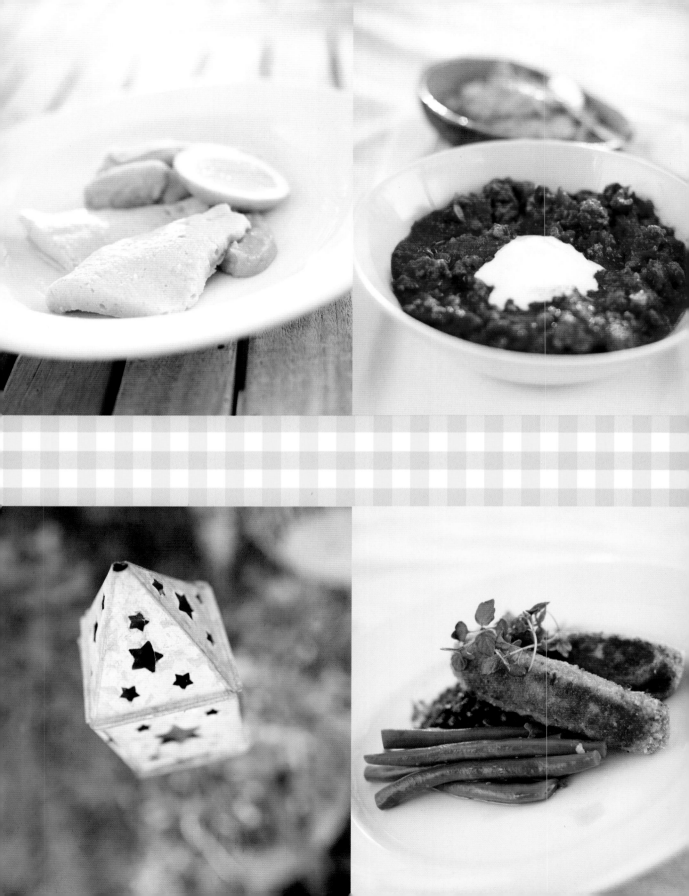

Understanding swallowing

Prudence Ellis, Certified Practising Speech Pathologist

Hard to swallow

Many people with dementia experience difficulties with swallowing, known as dysphagia. These may develop in a variety of ways and can be unsettling for loved ones and carers. Early identification of swallowing difficulties is important and may assist with eating, drinking and ensuring adequate nutrition and hydration is maintained. It can also help maximise swallowing safety and ensure richer enjoyment of meals.

Difficulties can occur at any stage of swallowing, including putting food in the mouth, chewing, swallowing and when food travels to the stomach. These difficulties can range from mild to severe and may look like:

- trouble with chewing
- food spilling out of the mouth
- taking a long time to chew or eat a meal
- forgetting to swallow/holding food in the mouth
- spitting out pieces of food
- getting food 'stuck' in the throat
- coughing/throat clearing during or immediately after eating or drinking
- gurgly/wet voice just after eating/drinking
- refusing food or drinks
- having lots of food left in the mouth after a meal
- difficulty initiating a swallow
- overfilling of the mouth
- poor saliva management
- dry mouth
- regurgitation of undigested food.

It is important that people with dementia are observed regularly while eating, to help identify if any of these difficulties occur. If they aren't addressed quickly, the person could be at risk of coughing, choking, or inhaling food or drink into the lungs (called aspiration). This can lead to a chest infection or aspiration pneumonia.

If aspiration is occurring, people may or may not cough (the body's way of getting the food/fluid back out of the lungs). If people are not coughing when they aspirate, you might identify the aspiration later by noticing a high temperature or chesty cough, or diagnosis of a chest infection.

How to help

If someone is experiencing the symptoms above, it is important that you consult your local doctor and a speech pathologist. A speech pathologist is trained to identify problems with swallowing and the underlying physical and neurological causes. They will seek to ensure the person with dementia is able to enjoy food and drink as safely as possible.

This might involve suggesting modification to the texture and thickness of food and/or drinks, which can help to lessen difficulties swallowing or reduce symptoms of aspiration. Clinical standards have been developed to label and describe the levels of thickness of food and drink that can help people with dysphagia. These labels and descriptions vary around the world. In *Don't give me eggs that bounce*, the levels of thickness of fluids and texture modification of foods are those used in Australia.

Enjoying food with modifications

People with dementia or disability who require a modified diet do not have to miss out on the good stuff!

Texture-modified food may be recommended by a speech pathologist because regular food is placing a person at risk of aspiration. Most foods or drinks that are eaten every day can undergo simple modifications while maintaining enjoyment. The standard consistencies are:

- Regular—normal or unmodified food.
- Texture A—soft. Food that looks like 'normal' food, without the hard, crunchy or chewy bits (like a T-bone steak!). On this diet, people avoid toast, raw vegetables and nuts.

Examples of soft food are cooked vegetables, soft fruits, soft sandwiches and cereals. Anything dry, crumbly or flaky should be avoided.

- Texture B—minced and moist. Food that is finely cut-up (into 0.5 cm cubes) or run briefly through a blender (like bolognaise). Examples of minced and moist foods are cereal that is naturally soft or soaked until soft and tender, meats and vegetables that are finely diced.

- Texture C—smooth pureed. Food that is blended until smooth. On this diet, all food should be moist and blended in a food processor until no lumps remain. Examples of pureed foods include puree cereals, fruit and vegetables as well as gelled bread, smooth spreads and yoghurt.

Don't give me eggs that bounce features a range of innovative recipes and approaches to help people on modified diets continue to enjoy food and dining. For explicit information relating to a specific diet consistency, consult your speech pathologist.

When you need a stiff drink

If regular fluids place a person with dementia or disability at risk of aspiration, a speech pathologist may recommend that they drink thickened fluids.

Most drinks (even coffee or beer) can be thickened for safe consumption and this can often provide comfort to people as they continue to enjoy the experience of their favourite drink (see our 'Beverages' section). The standard consistencies are:

- Regular: normal, unmodified, thin fluids (from here on, regular fluids will be referred to as thin fluids to avoid confusion).

- Level 150—'mildly' thick fluids. These drinks have a slightly thicker consistency than fruit nectar. They should run off easily through a fork, leaving a thin film.

- Level 400—'moderately' thick fluids. These drinks are thicker again and resemble the thickness of honey. They should run off smoothly and slowly through a fork, with occasional drips.

- Level 900—'extremely' thick fluids. These drinks are thicker again, and resemble the thickness of pudding or yoghurt. They should run off a fork in a large 'plop'!

Thicken everything but be creative

It's important to remember that if the recommendation is for thickened fluids, all drinks and fluids should be thickened. This includes medications, supplements, sauces and soups. Even though some fluids (such as milkshakes and thickshakes) appear thick enough, they will melt in the mouth to a thin fluid.

Someone drinking moderately thick fluids (Level 400) should have moderately thick gravy on their meals (where appropriate), moderately thick soups and drink their medications with moderately thick fluids. If a dietitian has prescribed supplements for nutrition, these should be prepared according to the directions of the supplement and then thickened appropriately.

Having thickened fluids usually means no thin (regular) fluids at all, including in food. Ice cream, jelly and watermelon all contain thin fluids (when they melt in your mouth), so anyone using thickened fluids should avoid these.

When thickening fluids, read the instructions on the thickening powder for the quantity to use and directions. And be patient— sometimes it takes a few minutes to reach its required thickness.

Remember to be creative! Although someone needing thickened fluids cannot eat an ice block, you could thicken lemonade (or another drink) to the appropriate consistency and freeze it in an ice-block mould and you have created a safe, delicious treat.

Balancing safety and choice

Though a speech pathologist can provide recommendations to help support a person with dementia, it is always their choice (or their caregiver if decision-making capacity is an issue) to determine if they want to follow these recommendations. In some cases, people may agree to accept the risks and consequences of aspiration and make their own choices about what they eat and drink.

We advocate that this informed decision by the person with dementia (or carers), should always be respected to ensure quality of life is maintained and the people involved empowered.

Strategies to help with swallowing

People with dementia may at times do things with their food that seem peculiar to others. They may, for no obvious reason, refuse their food, spit out pieces, 'swoosh' drinks around their mouth, or play with their food.

A speech pathologist may be able to assist, but some behaviours may not be eliminated. In these cases, you could work with the speech pathologist and other health professionals to ensure a person's dignity, comfort and independence (where possible) is maintained. Work with the behaviours, not against them!

Some common problems and solutions are listed below, but should be personalised and implemented individually:

- Follow the directions in Chapter 2 for ensuring the environment is optimised for positive dining—this is crucial!

- Spitting out pieces of food—consider providing a napkin on which to place the food.

- Encourage the person with dementia to feed themselves—even if this means putting food on a spoon and guiding their hand to their mouth. This can help them swallow more effectively.

- Ensure they see the food as it is brought to their mouth—remind them of what they are eating.

- If the person is keeping lots of food in their mouth after they have swallowed:

  > offer sips of drink between mouthfuls of food.

  > encourage them to swallow again (without any more food) before taking another mouthful.

- Difficulty chewing:

  > allow more time for them to eat their meal

  > consult with a speech pathologist to determine if their diet is right for them.

- Overfilling their mouth:

  > consider portioning food into smaller servings

  > swap a dessert spoon, soup spoon or large fork for smaller cutlery, like a teaspoon and small cake fork

  > provide a companion for eating—or eat with them, and help them pace their meal by providing verbal prompts, like 'slow down'.

- Food spilling out of their mouth:

  > ensure positioning is optimised and that they are seated fully upright and not tilting to one side or another.

- Food getting stuck in their throat:

  > encourage them to swallow several times to allow the food to pass

  > consult with a speech pathologist to determine if their diet is right for them.

- Forgetting to swallow, not sensing food in the mouth and difficulty initiating a swallow:

  > provide verbal and tactile (gentle touch) prompts to remind them to swallow—this might include making conversation and asking questions about the food

  > alternate between food and drinks

> alternate between a teaspoon of food and an empty teaspoon

> try foods of different tastes, textures and temperatures (keeping in mind any food modifications that have been recommended)

> alternate between hot and cold food, or sweet and sour food

> if you need to feed the person (that is, they are unable to feed themselves at all), try applying light pressure with the back of a teaspoon on the middle of their tongue as you put the food in their mouth. This can sometimes help them close their mouths and remind them to swallow.

• Coughing/throat clearing/gurgly voice during or immediately after eating or drinking:

> these are signs of aspiration and you should consult your local doctor and a speech pathologist as soon as possible.

• Regurgitation of undigested food:

> liaise with your doctor—this may be a sign of gastrointestinal difficulties

> consult with a speech pathologist to determine if their diet is right for them.

• Dry mouth or difficulty managing saliva:

> ensure their mouth is empty after eating and drinking

> try mouth moisturisers (avoid sprays or mouthwash if recommended thickened fluids)

> try removing any leftover food or drinks with a sponge or swab.

Swallowing medications

Some people with dementia and dysphagia have difficulty swallowing medications. All people on thickened fluids should consume their medications with the appropriate fluids prescribed by a speech pathologist. This includes mixing soluble medications with thickened fluids (for example Movicol, Metamucil).

In some cases, medications may need to be crushed or broken into smaller pieces. Before doing so, always check with your pharmacist, as some medications cannot be crushed or broken (as this may affect the purpose of the tablet and cause side effects).

Don't rush, don't give up

Although there is a lot of clinical information involved in safe eating and drinking, there are important contributions we can all make to food enjoyment and safety.

One example is to not rush. People with dementia and dysphagia may need twice the amount of time (or more) to eat a full meal. And don't give up on finding ways to share the joy of food. Food is intertwined with emotion—always try to make food safe and appetising and enjoyable. You could make someone very happy!

For information on how to access a speech pathologist, see 'Contacts and resources'.

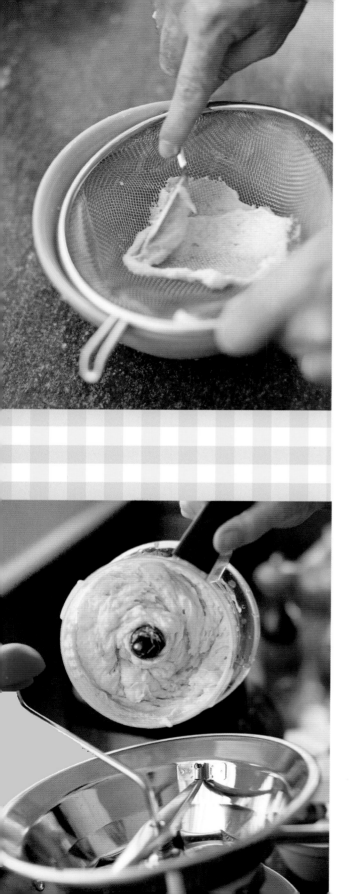

Preparing texture-modified food

Peter Morgan-Jones

Many people with dementia—and other conditions and disabilities—may be recommended texture-modified food and fluids and too often in the past this has led to reduced enjoyment of food. *Don't give me eggs that bounce* represents our passion to ensure, as much as possible, that this doesn't occur.

The greatest challenge with texture-modified food and fluids—such as smooth pureed, minced and moist, soft food and thickened fluids—is that these processes sometimes change the characterisation, integrity, presentation and colour of the food. All these factors are a catalyst for a person to lose their appetite which can result in weight loss, depression and apathy towards mealtimes.

Our hope is to inspire carers in thinking about ways to improve the look of texture-modified food at mealtimes. We also offer tips and contacts for obtaining appropriate items to enhance mealtimes for a person for whom texture-modified food or fluids are recommended.

Making sense of modifying

Many meals can be modified using basic kitchen appliances and utensils but this can affect the colour and translucency of the meal.

Most protein elements of a meal are brown, for example, roast beef. When this is blended with vegetables and gravy the whole meal takes on the colour of the meat—a light and unappetising brown colour. It can be more labour intensive but much more appealing, if all the meal's components can be modified separately and served on the same plate or served in smaller bowls. This way the different flavour profiles of each meal component can be appreciated.

Recipes and descriptions in this book are based upon the Australian standardised labels and definitions (Dietitian Association of Australia and The Speech Pathology Association of Australia Limited, 2007). It is important that these descriptions are understood and followed carefully in preparation of the food and fluids throughout this book. Recipes in this book have also been tested for consistency by a speech pathologist to ensure compliance.

How to achieve the perfect texture?

Most dishes can be converted to suit texture-modified food and fluids. It is important to establish a good understanding of the person you are caring for—their favourite meals in the past and their dislikes. This knowledge will be a great building block to a repertoire of tried and tested meals that are more likely to be eaten.

To help prepare texture-modified food, it is important to understand the consistency required and know the equipment that can achieve that consistency. The following table gives the consistencies of texture-modified foods, the equipment that can be used and examples of recipes in *Don't give me eggs that bounce*. As smooth pureed is a difficult consistency to achieve, in-depth recommendations follow later in this chapter.

'Our hope is to inspire carers in thinking about ways to improve the look of texture-modified food at mealtimes.'

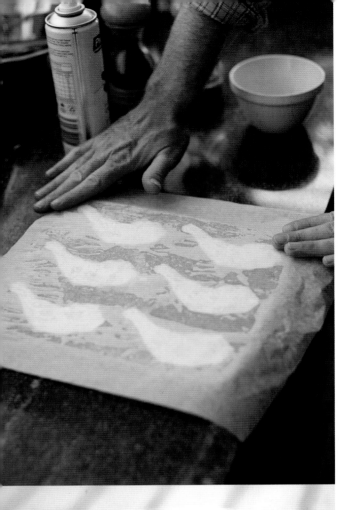

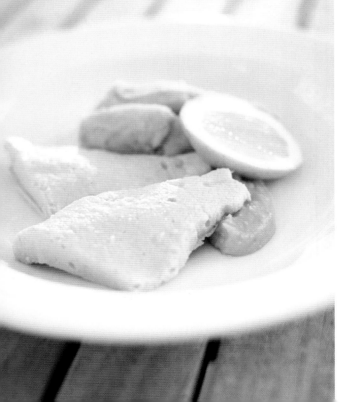

Consistency

Regular	
Texture A—Soft	
Texture B— Minced and Moist	
Texture C— Smooth pureed	

Description	Suggested equipment	Example recipes (see Index)
Normal foods—unmodified, including a variety of textures and consistencies as desired. These foods are sometimes referred to as a 'full' or 'normal' diet.		All foods and drink recipes in this book can be enjoyed.
Softer foods—meat cooked until tender and foods that are moist or that can be easily broken up with the back of a fork. Pieces should be no larger than 1.5cm in size. Crunchy, hard or dry foods must be avoided.	Food processor, stick blender, slow cooker	Chicken and corn soup with herb butter Risoni with bolognaise sauce Cottage pie Pizza soufflé
Food is moist and soft and diced into small pieces, no larger than 0.5cm in size. Food is textured and can be mashed with the tongue rather than chewed.	Food processor, stick blender, slow cooker, coffee grinder	Beef, shiraz and mushroom casserole Moroccan lamb Seafood chowder Boston baked beans
Pureed foods—all food should be blended until smooth and moist and be lump free. Foods may be slightly grainy due to their original form but this should be as smooth as possible.	Mouli, drum and conical sieves, cream whipper	Chicken drumstick satay with coconut rice and soy bean puree Smoked fish brandade Italian seafood and bean stew

For a detailed list of recommended foods and those to avoid for specific texture-modified diets, please contact your speech pathologist.

Pureed pastas, pulses, grains and rice

Many popular foods can be cooked so they are suitable for all levels of texture-modified diets. Here are some examples of preparing foods to be suitable for a smooth pureed diet.

Pasta

Risoni is a great pasta to use for a smooth pureed diet. It is a small, rice-like pasta. For best results:

Method

Blend a few batches in a coffee grinder until it resembles fine grit. Cook the risoni grit in salted water for 10 minutes or until cooked. Drain into a fine sieve and refresh under cold water to allow the starch to drain out. Then reheat with a little chicken or vegetable stock, olive oil and butter and season to taste.

Blend in a food processor until a smooth, thick consistency. Finely grated Parmesan cheese can be mixed in for taste and add more stock if the pasta is too dry.

Rice

A rice cereal or ground rice are the perfect starting point for making pureed rice. Use a good flavoured-stock when cooking the rice. See the 'Coconut rice' recipe in the 'Basics' section.

Method

Bring stock to the boil. Carefully pour in ground rice and stir until it thickens. Season to taste and add a small teaspoon of butter to improve the flavour.

Semolina and polenta

Semolina and fine polenta are also fantastic alternatives to potato for a main course. Semolina gnocchi and semolina pizza recipes are included in this book.

Grains

Grains and seeds are not recommended for smooth pureed diets as they may contain husks which are difficult to remove.

Soups and casseroles

Soups and casseroles tend to be the easiest of foods to turn into a texture-modified consistency. Thicker soups with lentils, cannellini beans, grains or potato are the easiest as they act as natural thickeners. If making soup and casserole, ensure any liquid is thickened to the appropriate consistency as recommended by a speech pathologist. Always create the meal then thicken appropriately afterwards.

A good tip is to drain the majority of liquid off first, retain to add later and blend the heavier mass first in a food processor or with a stick blender, adding the retained liquid slowly until the desired consistency of puree has been reached. It is much easier using this process than trying to thicken a large batch of runny soup.

Another tip is to keep food colours similar if making a soup. For example, if blending a tomato soup with peas, the soup will turn a brown colour, which may be less appetising.

Meat, modification and moulds

One of the innovations of *Don't give me eggs that bounce* is the inclusion of special recipes for preparing smooth pureed foods using moulds. This is especially important for meat, as preparing with a mould gives the person on a texture-modified diet dignity and makes it easier for them to identify the meal.

Fish, chicken and other meat require a more delicate process and work best blended with cream, seasoning and whipped egg white. The 'Salmon fillet' recipe in the 'Smooth pureed' section uses a method that can be applied to smooth pureed chicken and sausages. Another helpful recipe is 'Meatloaf modified' that uses a commercial thickener to 'set' the meatloaf to aid presentation.

Presentation is important when serving pureed meat. Try cooking in ramekins and then turn out the puree or try other shapes or moulds. Stockist for moulds can be found in 'Contacts and resources'.

Don't forget the vegetables

Vegetables can be split into three categories: hard, wet and salad.

Hard vegetables

To prepare hard vegetables, such as onion, broccoli and celery, it is always a good idea to cook the vegetables first in salted water, drain thoroughly and whilst hot, pass through a mouli or ricer with seasoning, a little cream and/or butter. For a smooth pureed diet, ensure they are lump-free. In the 'Basics' section you will find a large selection of vegetable purees.

Some hard vegetables with a watery content, such as parsnip, pumpkin and carrot, are best cooked in the same pot with 25 per cent peeled, diced potato. The potato acts as a binder and absorbs the liquid content.

Wet vegetables

Wet vegetables have a large water content, such as spinach, squash and zucchini. It is best to cook them and then squeeze out all the moisture. Then continue cooking with cream and seasoning, reduce the mixture in a pan and puree in a food processor. For a smooth pureed diet, ensure they are passed through a mouli or ricer until lump free.

Salad vegetables

Salad vegetables, such as cucumber, lettuce and tomatoes, are all best prepared by turning into a liquid (using a food processor) and thickened using commercial thickeners.

Method

Blend the vegetable in the food processor. Use a sieve to remove any seeds or skin/peel. Mix in the thickening agent (following instructions on the container) to achieve the consistency required—see 'Tomato jelly' in the 'Mid meal' recipe section.

And now for dessert

There are many desserts that are already ideal for a smooth pureed diet without alteration, including pannacotta, mousse, smoothies and thick milkshakes. Not so obvious is what can be done with bread, cakes, scones and biscuits—even for a smooth pureed diet.

Softened bread and cake

Let me share my favourite technique for softening bread, cakes and sponges. The method is called soaking and can be used with any sponge or porous food. This includes slices of bread (no crust, good quality sourdough works best), scones (sliced in half first), Madeira cake, sponge cake, biscuits, jam rolls, banana bread (no nuts), English muffins and crumpets.

The good thing about this method is that it has zero impact on the original taste of the food. This is not the case using gelatine.

Method

Soaking solution: to get started, use 1 tbsp Nestlé ThickenUp Clear whisked into 200ml water (multiply the amount to suit the requirements, for example 1 litre water to 5 tbsp). Ensure there are no hard and crusty parts to the food or nuts or seeds. Slice the food so that it is no more than 1cm thick. For scones it works best if you use a lighter scone recipe without butter in the ingredients.

Place the item into the solution and leave until it softens to the touch, or when a skewer is inserted easily. Softening time varies for each product, from one to 10 minutes. Bread takes about 30 seconds to 1 minute to soak through.

Scones work best if you immerse them quickly into the water, just as it has the ThickenUp Clear whisked into it, before it starts to thicken. This also is the case with any denser sponge-type foods.

When the soaked food feels soft, carefully remove with a slotted spoon and place on serving side plate. You can scrape away excess soaking liquid with a palette knife before plating. It can be covered and refrigerated for two hours minimum or serve at a later time that day.

Serve with seedless jam and, for the scones, whipped cream, for a memorable smooth pureed high tea!

Sponges can also be soaked in a jelly—this is ideal for a smooth pureed diet and is similar to the base of a trifle. The 'Cherry jelly cheesecake' in this book is an example of a great puree-friendly recipe.

Pureed sandwiches are a great idea, and look (and taste) like a regular sandwich—sourdough is more porous and works best. Follow the directions above for the first piece of bread. Place puree filling on top and repeat with top layer of bread, cover and refrigerate. Serve within two hours. Puree fillings can be:

- ham or chicken blended with butter and cream to form a paste

- sieved, cooked egg—push cooked egg through stainless steel sieve and fold in mayonnaise and seasoning.

It doesn't take long to get the hang of this softening method, just ensure there are no nuts, seeds, coconut strands or pieces of fruit in the food to be soaked.

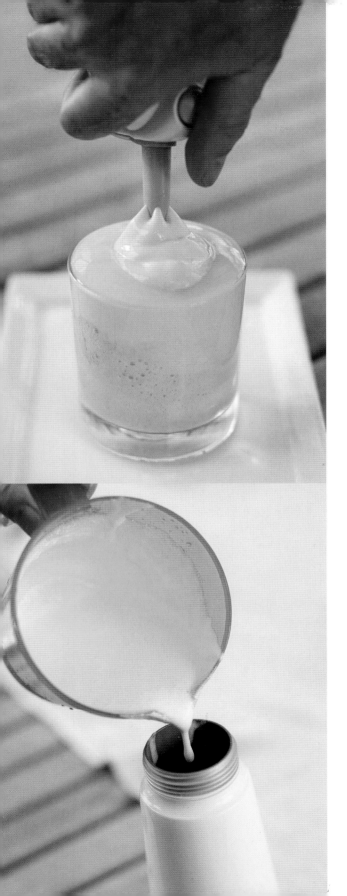

Wonderful world of thickening fluids

There is virtually no limit to the drinks that can be thickened. Fruit juices (without pulp), soft drinks, tea and coffee, wine and beer can all be enjoyed as thickened drinks. Commercially available thickening agents should be used to ensure that the right consistency is achieved in both hot and cold drinks. The stockists for all products can be found in the 'Contacts and resources' section.

'Most dishes can be converted to suit texture-modified food and fluids.'

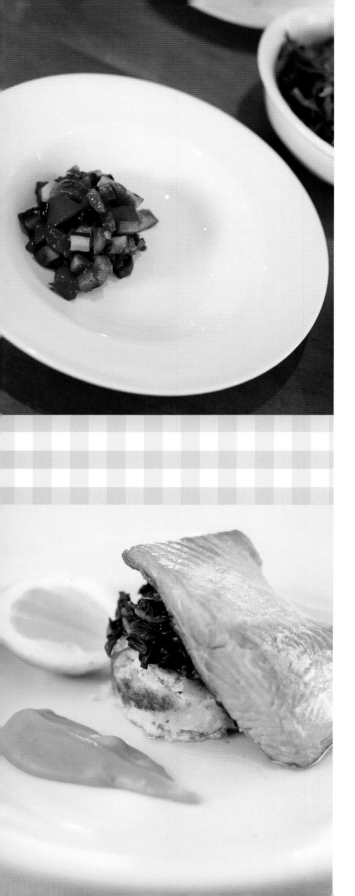

Plating, presentation and the power of our senses

Peter Morgan-Jones

Senses and food enjoyment

Our five senses—sight, taste, touch, hearing and smell—play an important role in making us feel hungry, helping us understand what we are eating and influencing how much we enjoy the meal.

This is as true for a person living with dementia or other disability as it is for anyone. And yet too often food is served to these communities without regard for the natural role of our senses. Is it any wonder that, sometimes, poor appetite and frustration at mealtime can occur?

Changing this is at the heart of what I do as an Aged Care Food Ambassador and is the passion behind *Don't give me eggs that bounce*. Spending time sharing food with many wonderful people with dementia has convinced me of the importance of taking seriously the mainly self-evident role of our senses in food enjoyment.

10,000 reasons for great food smells

Smell is one of the most important senses for stimulating the brain in relation to food—in fact, our appreciation of flavours actually comes from our sense of smell. The human brain can register 10,000 different odours at any one time and this process starts before we are even born. It is these triggers that are so important, particularly for people with dementia.

A long forgotten smell—such as the aroma of a sweet shop or baking bread—could be a trigger for appetite in someone who shows little interest in food.

The importance of smell is underscored, a little sadly we think, by the fact that some aged care services, where prepared food is shipped in to be reheated on site, have started installing 'scent clocks' to produce aromas at mealtimes to compensate for the lack of smell emanating from the food.

Tantalising our taste buds

Of course, it goes without saying that taste plays a crucial role in the dining experience. The five taste sensations are sweet, salty, bitter, sour and umami. Sweet taste is a pleasurable sensation, salty taste improves the flavour of food and bitter taste is a primeval protection against poisonous and inedible foods. Sour taste aids digestion and umami taste is a natural monosodium glutamate (MSG).

Getting to know a person's preferences and taste palette can help improve their dining experience and increase the enjoyment they get out of their food. We know that tastes can diminish and change with ageing and even more so with dementia. At age 30 a person has 245 tastebuds but this falls to about 80 by the time a person is 70-years-old.

Hungry eyes

Food that doesn't look appealing often goes uneaten. Presentation is an important aid to appetite. When we look at food our eyes take in the colour, gloss, physical form and the mode of presentation, such as the crockery and cutlery.

Other sight factors, especially important for an older person or someone living with dementia, are good lighting and distinguishable plates, like those with borders that 'frame' the food and draw the diner's eye to their food.

Eating with your ears

Sound often contributes negatively to the dining experience in the form of distracting noises. See Chapter 2 for great advice on this topic. The link between sound and food is the subject of an emerging field of research called 'neurogastronomy' which is exploring the ways in which music and other background noises stimulate the dining experience.

If you need convincing, next time you are on an aeroplane, take some noise cancelling earphones. Start eating your meal with the headphones on and then, midway through the meal, remove them and continue eating. The noise of the plane affects the 'flavour' of the food.

What's touch got to do with it?

The final sense to play an important part in the dining experience is touch. The feel of the food we eat and the cutlery and crockery we use to eat it influences the way we receive it. For example, if you have a barbecue and serve the meal on a paper plate with a plastic knife and fork, the meal will not taste the same as it would if it were served on china with a metal knife and fork.

Beautiful presentation is possible

Appetite often begins in the mind and poorly presented food may stop people feeling hungry. How food is plated, or arranged on the plate and garnished, figures deeply in one's reaction to it. It even affects how we think the food tastes. The good news is that great presentation is not that difficult, even for busy carers at home. Here are a few food presentation tips to help you begin to understand this incredibly important aspect of gourmet cooking.

A work of art

A plate of food is like a painting and the rim of the plate is the frame. This does not mean that you have to spend as much time arranging the plate as Rembrandt did painting a portrait, but it does mean that you need to think a little like an artist and strive for a pleasing arrangement. A plate that's too elaborate can be as bad as one that's too careless.

Create a clock. If you're serving protein, starch and vegetables, arrange the three items according to the face of a clock, with starch at 10, meat around 2, and vegetables below 9 and 3. Make sure one of the items acts as a focal point on the plate.

Balance and colour

Select foods and accompaniments that offer variety and contrast, while at the same time avoiding combinations that are awkward or jarring. A 'jarring' example is fish and chips with beetroot puree and lemon. A better example would be peas, chips and fish with lemon.

Two or three colours on a plate are usually more interesting than just one. Visualise the combination: poached chicken breast with cream sauce, mashed potatoes, and steamed cauliflower. Not too good? Or how about roast chicken, french fries and corn? Not quite so bad, but still a little monotonous. Now picture roasted red peppers, grilled stuffed chicken breasts on herbed orzo, with a drizzle of green pesto. Visually more appealing!

Many hot foods—especially meats, poultry, and fish—have little colour other than shades of brown, gold or white. It helps to select vegetables or accompaniments that add colour interest—one reason why green vegetables are so popular.

Getting into good shape

Another food presentation tip is to plan for variety of shapes and forms as well as of colours. For example, you probably do not want to serve Brussels sprouts with meatballs and new potatoes. Green beans and mashed potatoes might be better choices for accompaniments.

Cutting vegetables into different shapes gives you great flexibility. Carrots, for example, can be adapted to nearly any plate, by cutting them into a dice, rounds or sticks (batons or julienne).

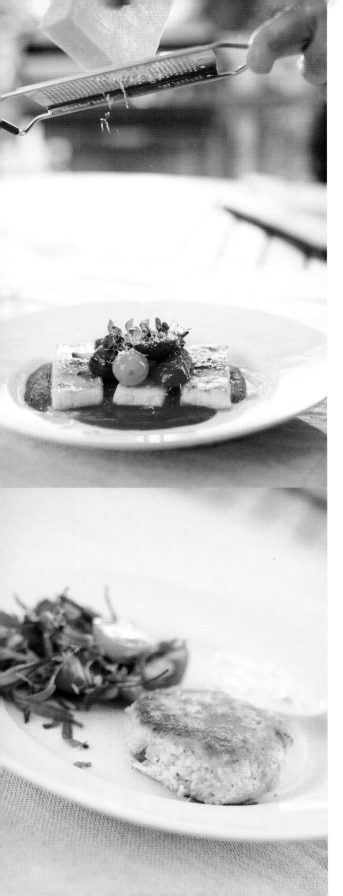

Textures talk too

Though not usually included in food presentation advice because they are not strictly visual considerations, textures are as important in plating as in menu planning. This is even more important for people with dementia or disability and their carer when preparing texture-modified food.

Here are some ideas for presenting texture-modified food:

- Blend meat separately from vegetables.

- Serve in separate, small bowls.

- Use small cups as a mould for potato or thickened proteins. Tip: Put plastic wrap in the cup first, add food and invert cup onto plate, then remove the plastic wrap.

- Use a serving spoon to create quenelles (egg shaped scoops). Tip: plastic wrap the spoon as this can stop potato sticking.

- Use cutters as rings to place pureed food into, removing cutter after food is formed.

- Use piping bags to pipe meat into a sausage shape onto plate, or to create potato swirls.

- Use a mould for pureed meals to give them a shape and contours.

Finally, flavours

You can't see flavours, either, but this is one more factor you must consider when balancing colours, shapes, and textures on the plate.

Hopefully we have inspired you to find enjoyment in plating and presenting food— we're confident it will make a positive difference for your mealtimes.

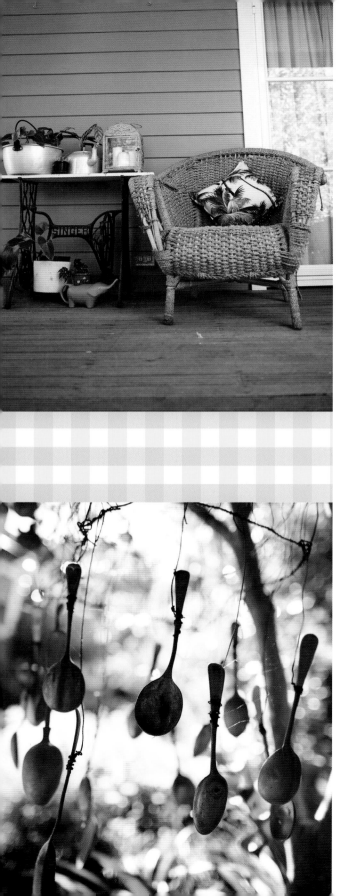

Caring for the carer

Danielle McIntosh and Emily Colombage

Caring for someone requires emotional and physical strength. So it is important that carers look after their own health, including nutritional and hydration needs. Many simple steps can support healthy eating and drinking, along with time-savers to assist in being an effective carer.

Be mindful of what you eat

Carers may rush through the day without a thought for themselves. Some find because of stress they forget to eat, while others eat more than they need to as a way of coping. Be aware of what you are, or are not eating. Aim for three meals a day and healthy snacks in between if you feel hungry. Remember to drink lots of fluid, water is best.

Sitting down and sharing a meal with the person with dementia can provide many benefits, as well as ensuring that you take time to eat. Even providing physical help for a person to eat their meal, does not mean you should not eat at the same time. Making the meal a social occasion and maintaining familiar routines can emotionally support the person being cared for.

Of course the meals contained in *Don't give me eggs that bounce* are for everyone—even the texture-modified meals! Rather than cook another meal for yourself, share the same meal. But, a word of caution: our meals have been created to be high in energy (calories/kilojoules) and high in protein. If you are watching your weight, needing to lose weight or on a specific diet restriction (such as low salt, low fat), always having the same meals might not be appropriate.

Time and energy savers

As a carer you have many responsibilities and tasks, including shopping, cooking and cleaning. Work simplification and energy conservation techniques can be useful to help you balance and achieve all that needs to be done.

When compiling the recipes in this book, attention was paid to simplifying steps so they are as easy as possible. Cooking a complicated meal is not something you would want to do every day, although many people find cooking relaxing!

Here are some useful work simplification tips to try:

Write a list and prioritise

When juggling responsibilities and tasks it is understandable that some things might be forgotten or are done late. Unfortunately, when you realise this has happened, you may come down hard on yourself and a vicious cycle begins. The more you try to do, the more you may get behind, the worse you feel. All of this can impact on the important task of preparing tasty, nutritious food for your loved one and yourself.

To help, a good idea is to write a list of everything that needs to be done—each hour, each day, each week, each month. Once you have done your lists, go through each task and prioritise them. Just because something may be prioritised as 'not vital' does not mean it should be forgotten. It is an opportunity to sit and look at what is important and what can be done if time allows. Asking a friend or family member to go through your list and give feedback on your priorities can also be helpful.

Get your shopping into shape

Grocery shopping can be a stressful and unpleasant experience for busy carers. Many comment that they do it as quickly as possible and then find they've forgotten something.

Writing a shopping list is a good routine to get into. Have a piece of paper handy in the kitchen so that when you run out of an item you can add it to your list. A note near the door or in the car to remind you to bring the shopping list can be useful too!

Many supermarkets have store layout maps which list all the items in each aisle. Using the map can save time and energy in finding everything you need.

If doing the shopping provides you with an opportunity to get out of the house and spend some time on yourself (a great idea), then this next tip is not for you. It takes just as much time and energy doing a weekly shop as it does a fortnightly shop. So, why not do a big shop less frequently—say fortnightly or monthly? Use your freezer to store perishables, such as fresh bread (take out the pieces you need so that they are fresh each day) and milk, or keep some long life milk in the cupboard as a back-up just in case.

Other tips to make grocery shopping easier include Internet shopping and home delivery. Most larger supermarkets offer online shopping with a home delivery service. You can do the shopping at any time that suits you. If the local supermarket does not provide online shopping, talk to them and see what service they could provide for you—remember if you are a loyal customer many businesses are keen to find ways to continue your patronage. Details of some online providers are available in 'Contacts and resources'.

Shopping is not just walking the aisles of your supermarket, it is also getting the groceries to your car or transport and then unpacking at home. Using a home delivery service may cost a little extra, but it can help save both time and energy. Some local supermarkets do provide this service free of charge. There are also companies that home deliver hot or frozen meals. See 'Contacts and resources'.

Canned and frozen food can be convenient

While *Don't give me eggs that bounce* champions great home-cooked meals, there is nothing wrong with using canned or frozen fruit and vegetables. Some frozen vegetables and rice also come in single-serve, microwavable packs to make it really easy. Another option some carers report as useful is using pre-made, packaged meals. Supermarkets have a wide selection of these and many healthier options. Even if you only use them occasionally, having something in the freezer ready-made for a tough day can be a good idea.

Cook in bulk and freeze

It takes almost the same amount of energy and time to cook a meal for one as it does for four. So cooking in bulk quantities can be good, as long as the meals can be frozen.

In this book, the recipes indicate if the dish is suitable for freezing. On your busy days or when those unexpected things happen, it will be a relief to know you can quickly pull meals out of the freezer and easily reheat.

Use technology if you can

If there is any group who need the time and energy saving benefits offered by 21st century technology, it is the devoted carers of the world.

And although our main focus is on food, anything that helps lessen carers' load will increase the likelihood of positive mealtimes. Not everyone is equally confident with technology but hopefully some of these ideas will help.

A dishwasher is great for taking care of the washing up and stacking dishes into the dishwasher after they have been used helps keeps the kitchen tidy. As an alternative, keep water and detergent in a sink so you can wash up as you go and leave items in the drying rack rather than drying yourself. Encourage the person with dementia to wash up or to help you dry up. It can be a great opportunity to spend time together and two pair of hands are better than one!

Internet banking helps to manage finances and bills and avoid the queues as well. Most banks and financial institutions offer online bill paying or automatic direct debit. Utilities such as water, electricity, gas and council rates can often be paid through regular automatic deductions. This can take the stress out of remembering to pay bills.

Phone or computer reminders can be very convenient, if you are confident using

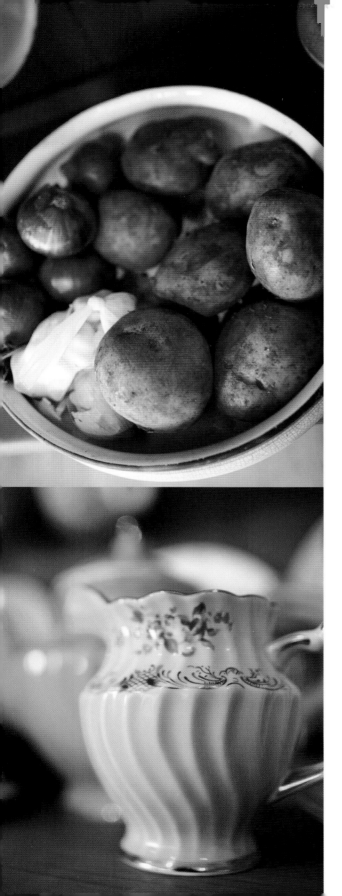

computers. You can transfer your task list into the reminders section of your email program or similar. These reminders can be set to alert you when they are due and you can tick them off when completed. For most tasks you only need to enter them once and set them as a recurring event. If computers are not your thing, then use a calendar on the wall to remind you of what is due and when.

There are many smart phone or tablet applications (apps) that are designed to help us stay organised and informed and so if you are confident with these technologies, they may further streamline your day. Let us know your favourite technology tips.

Home delivered meals may be useful

There will be times that you may feel unwell or that you are going to be very busy with appointments/commitments and cooking a meal may be one too many jobs to fit into the day. There are organisations and companies that can provide meals and home deliver them to your door. Some are delivered hot, ready to eat, while others need to be reheated. While cooking fresh food at home is always best, it is good to have some options to call on when you need them. See 'Contacts and resources'.

Share *Don't give me eggs that bounce* with friends and family

Family and friends not sure what they can do to help you? Perhaps they can read this book and learn about how to support a person with dementia and in turn support you. Or they could make some of the recipes in this book and host a dinner party, or bring food over.

Also, there are organisations, support groups and other books available to support carers in their role. See 'Contacts and resources' and for books, hammondcare.com.au.

Peter Morgan-Jones is arguably Australia's leading aged care chef and he has caringly created 118 original recipes for *Don't give me eggs that bounce.* Beginning with regular meals and snacks for throughout the day and moving on to texture-modified dishes, all the recipes aim to maximise taste and enjoyment, particularly for older people and people living with dementia or disability.

The texture-modified food and fluids are a key aspect of the innovation of *Don't give me eggs that bounce* and of Peter's passion to bring amazing taste and presentation to all people, regardless of age or eating function.

Alongside the usual inclusions of ingredients and method, you'll see symbols to indicate the texture-modified food or fluids for which the recipe is suitable. These guidelines are the result of our clinical testing of each recipe.

For example, if a recipe has the symbols R, T, S, MM and Th3, it means the recipe is suitable for people on regular, soft and minced and moist diets and those who can have thin fluids right through to those who need their fluids extremely thick.

Recipes

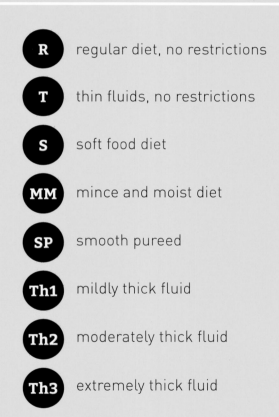

R regular diet, no restrictions

T thin fluids, no restrictions

S soft food diet

MM mince and moist diet

SP smooth pureed

Th1 mildly thick fluid

Th2 moderately thick fluid

Th3 extremely thick fluid

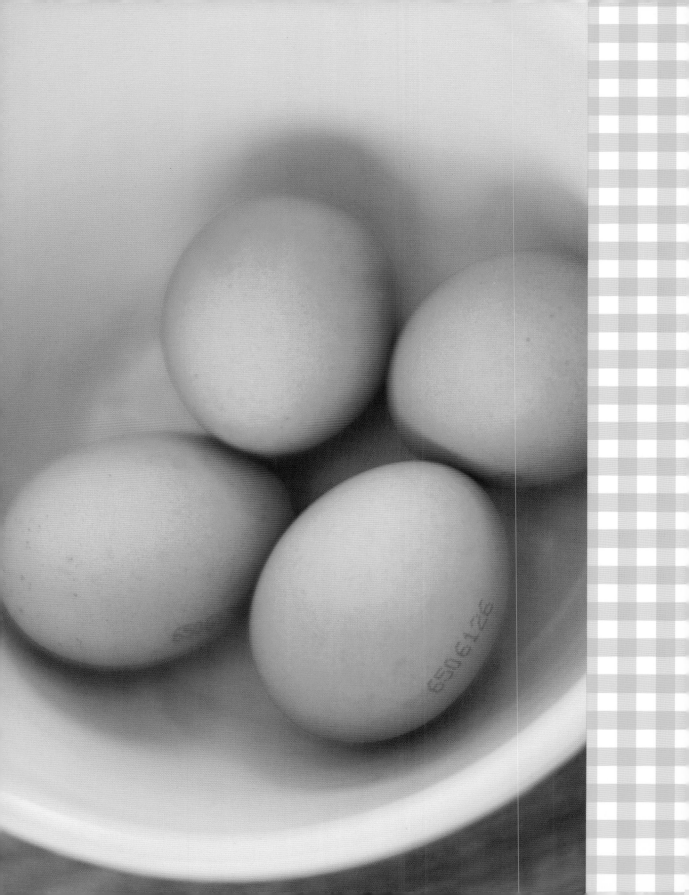

Breakfast

Breakfast is sometimes described as the most important meal of the day and it is especially important for vulnerable people with health challenges. These tasty recipes will help start the day well with colourful new ideas and comforting favourites.

Toasted muesli

Serves About 15 (1.5kg of muesli) • **Prep** 10 mins • **Cook** 5 mins

Dry Ingredients
3½ cups rolled oats
1½ cups wholegrain
   quick oats
1 cup shredded coconut
½ cup pepita
1½ cup chopped
   walnuts/almonds
1 cup dried cranberries
1 cup currants
3 tbsp cinnamon ground

Melt Ingredients
¾ cup coconut oil
¾ cup honey

Mix the dry ingredients together. Pour in the melt ingredients and combine.

Place in a microwave pot and microwave on high for 2 minutes. Remove and stir. Rest for 5 minutes.

Repeat previous step. Serve each portion with ½ cup of milk or yoghurt.

Tips: ~Allow the left over muesli to completely cool before placing in an airtight container. ~The muesli can keep up to 2 weeks in an airtight container in a cupboard/pantry.

(R) (T)

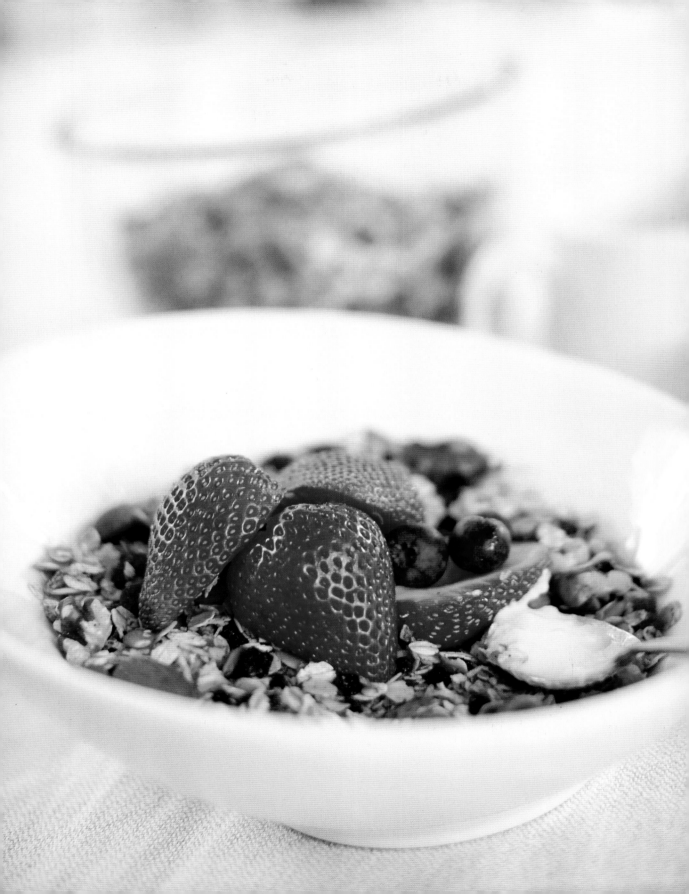

Bircher muesli

Serves 2 • **Prep** 10 mins • **Cook** 5 mins

1 cup rolled oats
Juice from ½ lemon
100g frozen mixed berries
¾ cup orange juice,
    freshly squeezed
1 cup plain natural yoghurt
2 tbsp honey
1 Granny Smith apple,
    grated with skin on
1 tbsp flaked almonds
(omit for soft diet)
¼ tsp cinnamon

Place rolled oats in a bowl. Squeeze the lemon and orange juice into the bowl. Stir to soften the oats. Cover and leave in refrigerator overnight.

In the morning, add honey, yoghurt, apples and cinnamon into the muesli. Mix well. Serve and top with berries and flaked almonds (omit for a soft diet).

Tips: ~Poached fruit can be added as well. ~Defrost mixed berries overnight on an absorbent paper in the fridge.

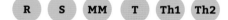

Bircher muesli (modified)

Serves 1 • **Prep** 1 mins • **Cook** 1 mins

1 cup rolled oat flakes
1 cup apple juice
100g (½ cup) yoghurt,
    vanilla or natural
4 small scoops
    Gelea Instant
Pinch of cinnamon

Place the rolled oats in a coffee grinder (see 'Helpful kitchen equipment') and grind until a firm meal is reached. Remove and place in a container with the apple juice and seal and leave overnight in the refrigerator.

Remove from the refrigerator and place in a small stainless steel saucepan, add the Gelea Instant (see 'Contacts and resources') and stir through the oats, place onto heat and bring to simmer and stir continuously for 1 minute.

Remove from heat and place into serving bowl. Allow to cool and with a small whisk fold through the yoghurt and cinnamon until it is all thoroughly mixed together. Serve with a puree banana or berry compote (see Basic recipes) if desired.

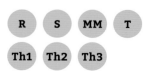

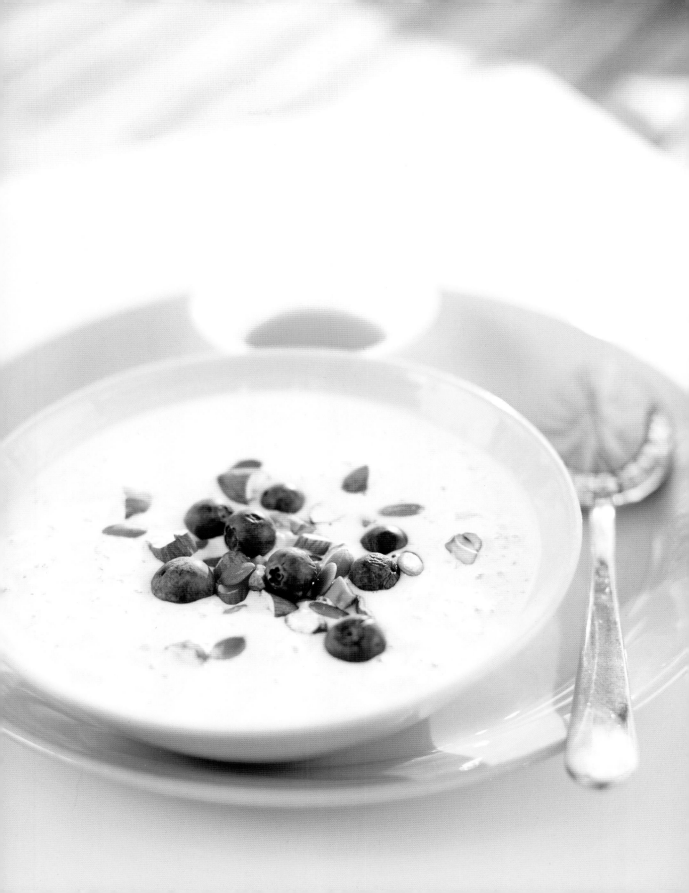

Honey and banana Weetbix

Serves 1 • **Prep** 5 mins

1½ Weetbix, crumbled
1 small banana
½ cup thickened cream
½ cup hot milk
1–2 tsp honey

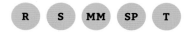

Place crushed Weetbix in a small bowl. Pour over hot milk and allow Weetbix to soften (if on a smooth pureed diet ensure it is thoroughly soaked until smooth).

Blend banana, cream and honey using a blender. If on a smooth pureed diet, strain mixture through a sieve to ensure it is lump free. Add to Weetbix and stir.

Tips: ~Extra can be made and stored in the fridge for later in the day. ~Vanilla essence is also a delicious accompaniment to the milk. ~A high-energy recipe.

Banana and coconut porridge

Serves 2 • **Prep** 5 mins • **Cook** 15 mins

1½ small bananas
  (mashed well for
  minced and moist diet)
1 cup rolled oats
1½ cups full cream milk
½ cup water
¼ cup coconut milk
2 tbsp sultanas
½ cup long shredded coconut
  (omit for soft or mince
  and moist diets or use
  desiccated coconut)
2 tsp brown sugar (or honey)
Salt to taste

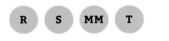

In a small, heavy-based saucepan, add milk, water, rolled oats, bananas, sultanas and half of the shredded coconut. Bring to the boil. Once boiled, turn down to simmer and cook for 10–12 minutes.

(Omit the following step for minced and moist or soft diets). Meanwhile, toast the remaining shredded coconut by placing it under the grill until golden brown. Add the coconut milk to the porridge until correct consistency is reached. Remove from heat.

Distribute into bowls and sprinkle with brown sugar and finish with coconut (regular diet). If you are cooking this for a soft or minced and moist diet, sprinkle untoasted coconut on top and mix thoroughly.

Tips: This can also be served with poached pears, apricots or pineapple.

Ricotta hot cakes with banana and vanilla honey

Serves 2-3 • **Prep** 10 mins • **Cook** 10 mins

250g ricotta cheese
125ml full cream milk
2 large eggs, separated
100g plain flour
1 tsp baking powder
1 pinch salt
2 tsp rice bran oil
250g banana, sliced
Drizzle of vanilla honey
   (see below)
Icing sugar, sifted

Vanilla Honey
2 tbsp honey
¼ tbsp vanilla essence

Put ricotta, milk and egg yolks into a bowl and mix well to combine. Stir in the flour, baking powder and salt and gently whisk to make a smooth batter. Beat the egg whites until foamy and then fold them into the ricotta mixture. Peter says: 'This isn't hard work, just whisk by hand.' Heat the oil in a large frying pan and spoon a heaped dessert spoon of batter into the pan. Cook the hot cakes for about 1 minute until golden and then flip them over and cook for another minute. Keep the cooked hot cakes warm. Continue making more hot cakes with remaining batter.

Serve with sliced banana and a drizzle of vanilla honey. Sprinkle icing sugar over the top.

Tip: This dish is a great source of calcium.

R   T

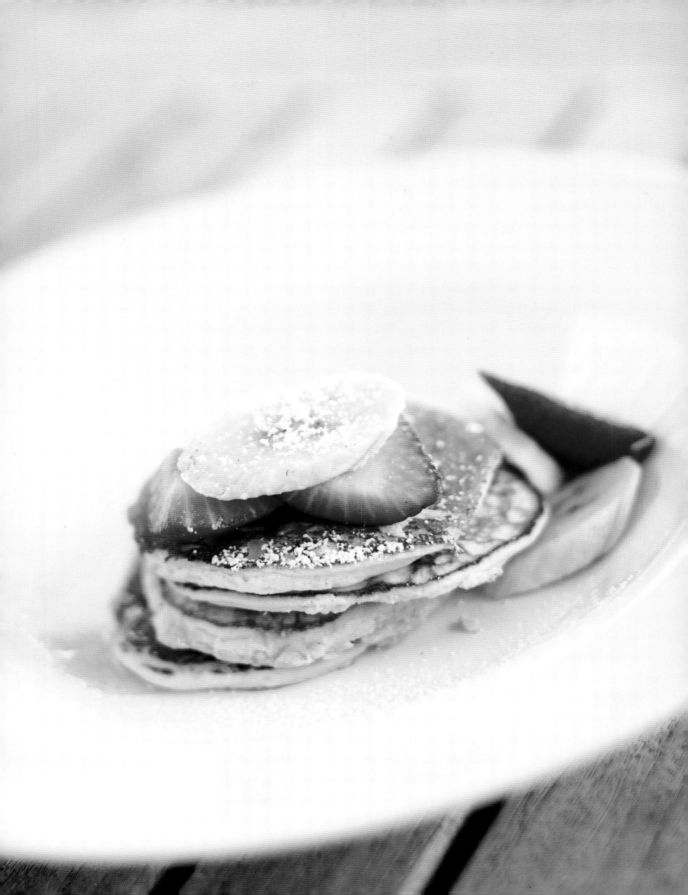

Baked ricotta and prune pot

Serves 2-4 • **Prep** 1 mins • **Cook** 15 mins

100g pitted prunes
120ml full cream milk
120ml thickened cream
4 eggs, lightly beaten
150g ricotta
3 tsp caster sugar

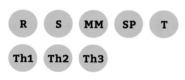

Preheat oven to 130°C. Grease 4 ramekins or Asian style bowls (125ml capacity) with butter.

Place the prunes in a food processor and blend until smooth, then pass the prunes through a sieve to remove any hard or stringy pieces of the pulp. Divide the prune puree into the 4 dishes.

Mix all the remaining ingredients together and pour carefully into the 4 dishes, on top of the prune puree. Cover each one with foil and place in a preheated oven for 40–45 minutes or until the baked ricotta has almost set in the centre of each ramekin.

Remove from oven and allow to cool before serving.

Tip: This can be prepared the night before and served the following morning for breakfast.

Pear with yoghurt

Serves 1 • **Prep** 3 mins • **Cook** 2 mins

100g cooked skinned pear,
   seeds and core removed
   (or use canned pears)
80ml pear juice
½ tsp fresh squeezed
   lemon juice
6 x small scoops Gelea
Instant (see 'Contacts
   and resources')
1 cup creamy vanilla
   yoghurt. For those on
   thickened fluids use
   vanilla Fruche (1 and
   a half tubs) or ensure
   yoghurt is lump free
   and thickened with
   a commercial thickener
Olive oil spray

Either poach fresh pears (see 'Basic recipes') or use canned pear slices. Measure 100g of the pear (drained weight) and place in a food processor with the pear juice and the lemon juice. Process until a smooth pureed is produced. Scrape all the pear puree from the bowl into a small stainless steel saucepan, add the Gelea Instant to the puree pear and stir.

Bring the pear to a simmer for 2 minutes, continuously stirring. Remove from the heat, then prepare the pear mould (see 'Contacts and resources') by spraying lightly with olive oil spray. Carefully pour the pear puree into the pear indentations in the mould. Place in refrigerator until firm.

Serve the pear with yoghurt.

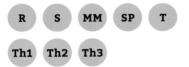

Israeli shakshuka

Serves 2 • **Prep** 10 mins • **Cook** 30 mins

½ tbsp olive oil
¼ medium brown onions,
  peeled and diced
½ clove garlic, mined
¼ red capsicum, diced
1 can (400g) diced tomatoes
1 tbsp tomato paste
1 pinch of chilli powder
½ tsp cumin
½ tsp paprika
2 eggs
¼ tbsp fresh chopped
  parsley (optional, as
  desired)
1 pinch of cayenne pepper
  (optional)
1 pinch of sugar
  (optional, to taste)
Salt and pepper to taste
4 bread slices (soft bread
  if required)–to serve

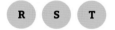

Heat a stainless steel pan and slowly warm the olive oil. Add the chopped onions and fry for 2-3 minutes until the onions are soft. Add garlic and continue to fry till fragrant.

Add capsicum and fry for 5–7 minutes until softened. Add tomatoes and tomato paste, stir until blended. Add chilli powder, cumin and paprika, stir well. Simmer mixture over medium heat for 5–7 minutes or until mixture starts to reduce. Add cayenne pepper and sugar (to taste) and season with salt and pepper to taste.

Crack the eggs, one at a time, directly over the tomato mixture. Make sure to space them evenly over the sauce. The eggs will cook 'over-easy' style on top of the tomato sauce. Cover the pan. Allow mixture to simmer for 10 minutes, or until the eggs are cooked and the sauce has slightly reduced. Peter says: 'Keep an eye on the pan to make sure the sauce does not reduce too much, which can lead to burning.'

Garnish with chopped parsley, if desired. Serve with warm crusty bread or pita that can be dipped in the sauce.

Tips: ~If you prefer the eggs to be more runny, let the sauce reduce for a few minutes before cracking the eggs on top. ~For a sweeter sauce, add more sugar. ~For a spicier sauce, add more cayenne pepper (be careful with the cayenne pepper, it is extremely spicy).

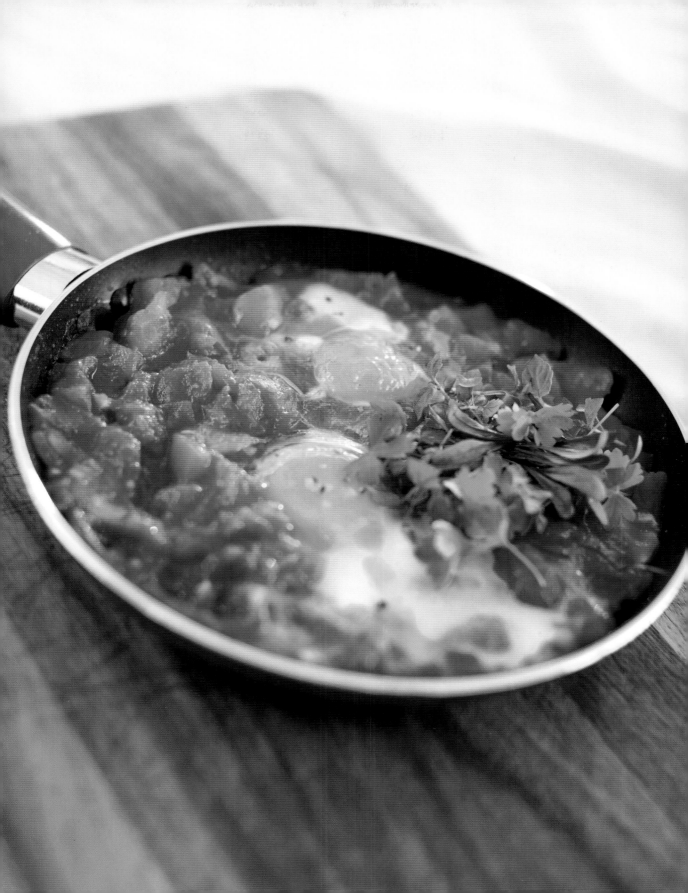

Classic scrambled eggs

Serves 1 • **Prep** 5 mins • **Cook** 15 mins

2 eggs
3 tbsp cream
2 tsp butter
Sea salt to taste
Ground white pepper
   to taste

For regular diet use two
pieces of sourdough or
multigrain toast. For soft
diet, use soft white or
wholemeal bread. For
minced and moist or
smooth pureed diet use
soaked bread.

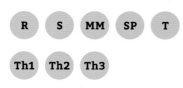

For regular or soft diet
Whisk the eggs together, add the cream and butter and
season with salt and pepper, place mix into a small
heat-proof bowl. Place the bowl over a pan of simmering
water and allow to cook really slowly using a spatula to
continuously stir the mixture.

Cook until the eggs begin to scramble–this should take
about 10–15 minutes. Serve on hot buttered toast for
regular diet. For soft diet, use soft bread (untoasted).

For minced and moist or smooth pureed diet
Remove the cooked eggs from the bowl and blend
with a stick blender. Serve with soaked bread–recipe
in Chapter 4.

Tips: ~Try flavouring the scrambled egg with smoked
salmon, just blend with the scrambled egg or sprinkle
in bacon dust or mushroom dust (see 'Basic recipes').
~For a smooth pureed diet, ensure it is lump free.
~Eggs are a great source of protein.

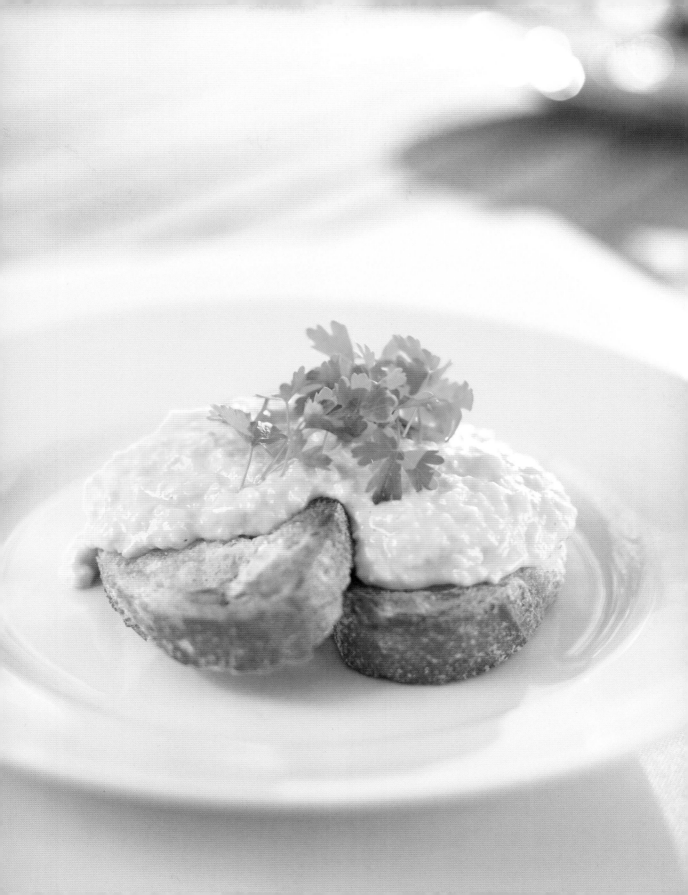

Perfect boiled egg with sourdough soldiers

Serves 1 • **Prep** 1 mins • **Cook** 10 mins

2 large eggs
2 slice sourdough toast,
    buttered, crust removed
    and cut into fingers.
Sea salt and pepper
    (to taste)

(R) (T)

Place the eggs in a small stainless steel pan and add enough cold water to cover them. Put the lid on the pan and place over high heat. When the water comes to the boil allow to boil for 1 minute, remove the pan from the heat and wait for 5 minutes.

After the 5 minutes, remove the lid and carefully remove each egg. Cut the top off each egg before serving in egg cups. Season with salt and pepper to taste and serve with sourdough soldiers.

Tips: Leave the eggs for 8 minutes in water for hard boiled, allow to cool before peeling.

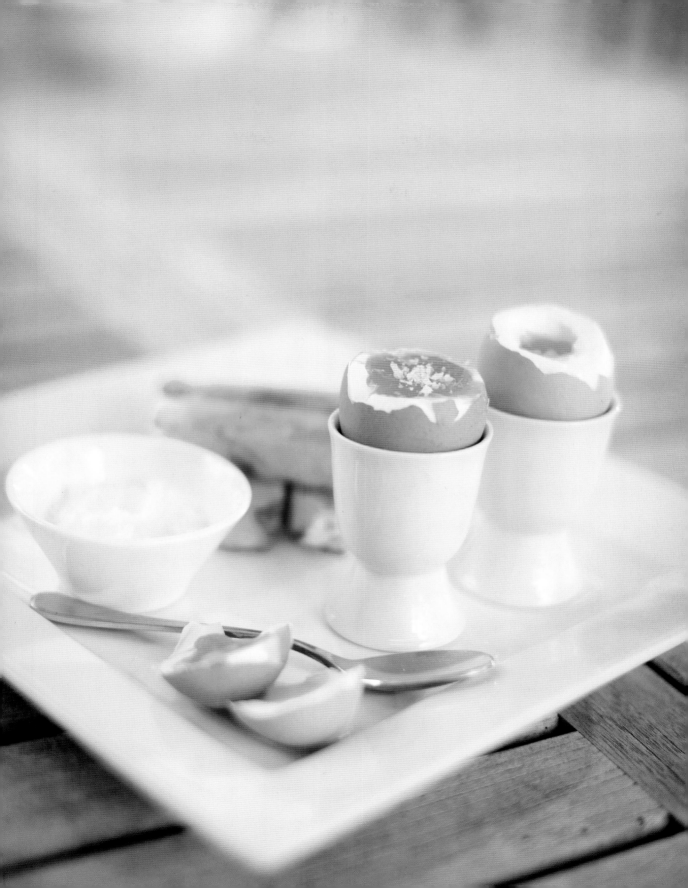

Leg ham and Gruyere and spinach croque monsieur

Serves 2 • **Prep** 5 mins • **Cook** 25 mins

Bechamel sauce
1 tbsp butter
1 tbsp plain flour
¾ cups milk
Pinch of salt
Pinch of freshly
  ground pepper
Pinch of nutmeg
½ cup Gruyere cheese,
  grated

Croque monsieur
4 large, thick slices of crusty
French or Italian bread
120g leg ham, sliced
1 cup wilted English
  spinach leaves
Dijon mustard
Butter (enough to spread
  on the bread slices)
¾ cup Gruyere cheese,
  grated
2 tsp olive oil

R T

Preheat oven to 180°C. Heat a small saucepan over low heat and melt the butter until it just starts to bubble. Whisk in flour and cook for 2 minutes, stirring until smooth. Slowly whisk in the milk, cooking until thick. Remove from heat. Season with salt, pepper and nutmeg. Stir in grated Gruyere.

Arrange the bread slices on a board, lightly brush one side of the slices with a little softened butter. Lightly spread the unbuttered side of two slices of bread with a little Dijon mustard. Distribute the leg ham and béchamel sauce evenly on top of the two slices (Dijon mustard side). Top each slice of bread with Gruyere cheese.

Heat 2 tsp of oil in a frying pan. Add the spinach leaves and stir-fry until wilted. When cooled, remove excess liquid from the spinach leaves by squeezing it. Place enough spinach on the bread slices to cover the toppings. Finish by placing the slice of bread with no fillings on top to complete the sandwich, with the buttered side facing outwards. Peter says: 'Both sides of the sandwich should have the buttered side on the outside.'

Heat a frying pan and place the sandwich (butter side) in and cook until lightly browned. Turn over and repeat on the other side. Place sandwich on a baking tray and put in oven for 5–10 minutes, or until cheese has started melting.

Serve immediately.

Tips: ~Serve with a poached egg for a great lunch meal.
~Can be served without the spinach, try tomato instead.

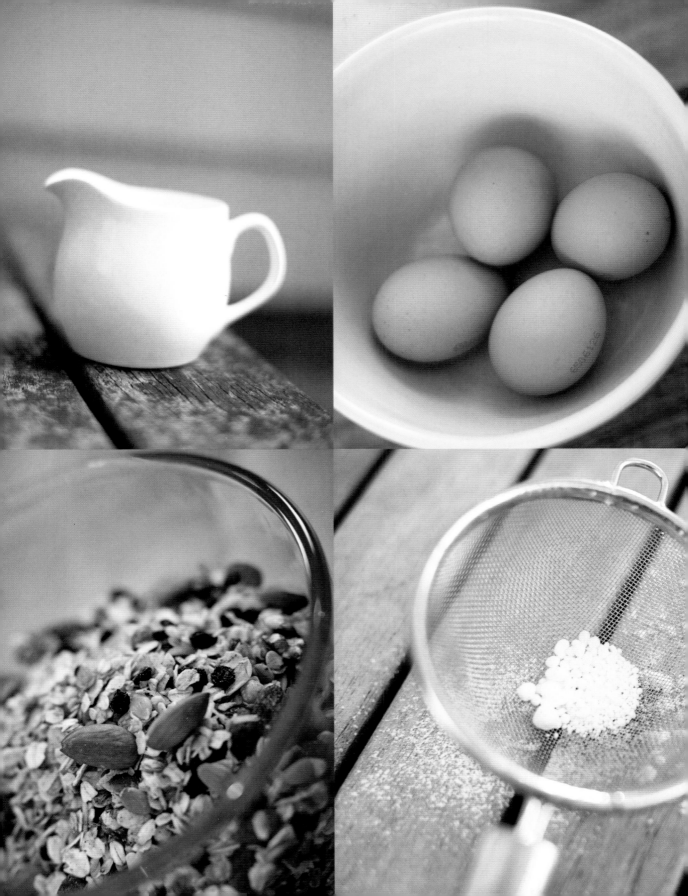

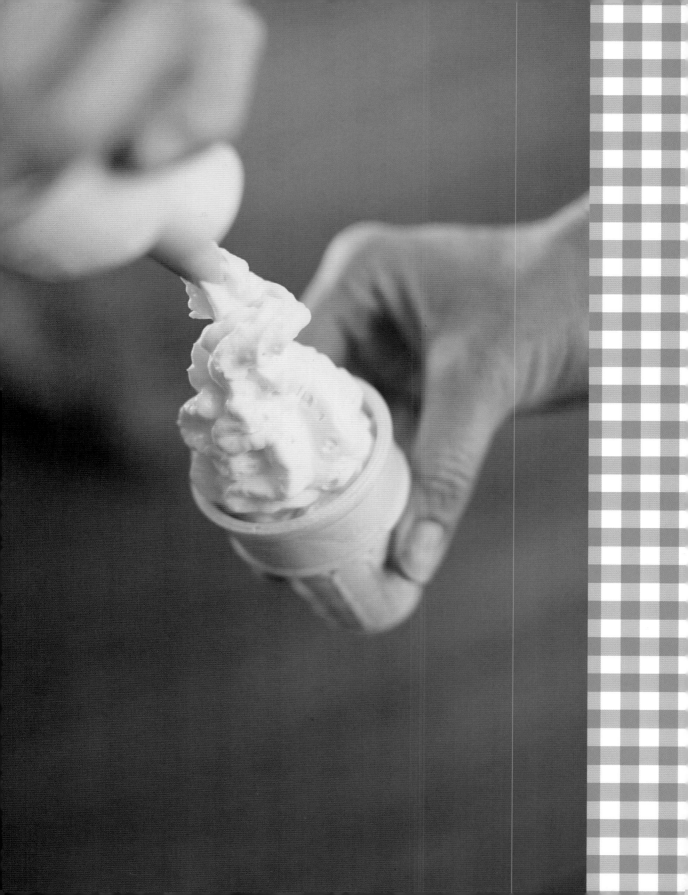

Mid meals

Mid meals (morning tea, afternoon tea
and supper) are important contributors
to overall nutrition across the day, especially
when someone can eat only a small meal
at one sitting (see Chapter 1).

Milk drinks are underrated for morning or
afternoon tea and are a great source of protein
and calcium. The milkshake recipes in this
section are all quick and easy. As well, you may
find it convenient to use a recipe to make up
a small jug in the morning, which can then be
served throughout the day.

High protein milkshake

Serves 2 • **Prep** 10 mins

250ml full cream milk
1 small banana frozen,
    peeled, cut into pieces
2 scoops ice cream
4 tbsp skim milk powder
1 tbsp maple syrup
    (optional)

Blend all ingredients together. If on a minced and moist/smooth pureed diet, strain through a sieve before serving. If on thickened fluids, thicken with a commercial thickener, following manufacturer instructions for required consistency.

Tip: Adding milk powder to milk or milkshakes is an easy and cheap way of boosting the protein and calcium of any recipe.

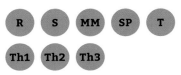

Strawberry almond milkshake

Serves 1 • **Prep** 3 mins

⅓ cup frozen strawberries
    (about 6 small strawberries)
⅓ cup extra creamy vanilla
    yoghurt
¼ cup full cream milk
1 tbsp of almond meal

Place all ingredients in blender and process until smooth. If on a minced and moist/smooth pureed diet, strain through a sieve before serving. If on thickened fluids, thicken with a commercial thickener, following manufacturer instructions for required consistency.

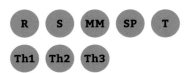

Peach, coconut and banana oatmeal smoothies

Serves 2 • **Prep** 5 mins

¼ cup rolled oats
½ banana
200g natural yoghurt
1 tsp vanilla honey (see
   recipe for hotcakes)
¼ cup coconut milk
¼ cup full cream milk
1 peach half (canned) or
   half a de-seeded fresh
   peach, peeled and sliced
Handful of berries, fresh
   or frozen (5–6) (optional)

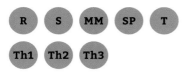

Place all ingredients in food blender, turn on to high and blend until smooth.

If on a minced and moist/smooth pureed diet, strain through a sieve before serving. If on thickened fluids, thicken with a commercial thickener, following manufacturer's instructions for required consistency.

Pour into 2 glasses and serve chilled.

Tip: ~Substitute coconut milk with milk if desired. ~If fresh berries are not available, you can substitute with frozen berries. ~When using frozen berries, remember to defrost them beforehand. ~Place them on absorbent paper in the fridge overnight.

Chocolate and peanut butter smoothie

Serves 2 • **Prep** 2 mins

½ small banana, chopped
½ cup (130g) plain yoghurt
½ cup (125ml) full cream
  milk
1 tbsp smooth peanut butter
3 tbsp chocolate
  topping/sauce
2 ice cubes

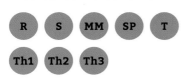

Blend all ingredients together in a blender. Divide into two glasses. Serve chilled.

If on a minced and moist or a smooth pureed diet, strain the smoothie through a sieve before serving. If on thickened fluids, thicken with a commercial thickener, following manufacturer instructions for required consistency. Ensure that ice cubes are fully crushed or melted before thickening.

Mango smoothie

Serves 2 • **Prep** 2 mins

½ small banana, chopped
1 small mango, skin and
  seed removed, flesh
  chopped
½ cup (130g) plain yoghurt
½ cup (125 ml) full cream
  milk
¼ cup of apple juice
  or pink grapefruit juice

Blend all ingredients together in a blender. Divide into two glasses, serve chilled. If on a minced and moist/smooth pureed diet, strain through a sieve before serving. If on thickened fluids, thicken with a commercial thickener, following manufacturer instructions for required consistency.

R S MM SP T
Th1 Th2 Th3

'...food that is appetising, tasty and nutritious with a special focus on energy and protein.'

French toast

Serves 2–4 • **Prep** 5 mins • **Cook** 2 mins (soft diet). 30 mins (minced and moist)

4 eggs
1 tsp sugar
½ tsp salt
250ml (1 cup) milk
2 slices of thick white
 bread—crusts can be
 removed (cut in half
 if serving 4)
1 tsp butter
Icing sugar to dust
1 punnet strawberries
 or 2 bananas

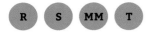

Regular
Break eggs into a wide, shallow bowl and beat lightly with
a fork. Stir in sugar, salt, and milk. Over medium-low heat,
heat a non-stick frying pan and add butter. Place the bread
slices, one at a time, into the bowl with the egg mixture,
letting slices soak up the egg mixture for a few seconds,
then carefully turn to coat the other side. Soak/coat only
as many slices as you will be cooking at one time.

Transfer bread slices to frying pan, heating slowly until
bottom is golden brown. Turn and brown the other side.
Serve French toast hot with butter and maple syrup and
a dusting of icing sugar.

Minced and moist
Prepare eggs as above. Ensure all the crust is removed
from the bread, break into 2cm squares and place in a
small, buttered Pyrex dish. Pour the batter carefully over
the bread and leave covered in fridge for 1 hour to absorb.

Preheat oven to 130°C. Cover the Pyrex dish with a lid
and cook in the oven for about 20–30 minutes or until the
custard has just set in the middle. Occasionally pull it out
and push the bread down into the batter, as it is likely
to float to the surface. When ready to serve, remove any
crusts or hard edges, dust with icing sugar and serve with
a crushed banana.

Tip: Try serving the French toast as a dessert with the
berry compote (see recipe), or with golden syrup, or
vanilla flavoured honey or with hulled strawberries or
banana, or custard.

Berowra ginger bread

Serves 12 • **Prep** 15 mins • **Cook** 1.5 hrs

2 x 400g can of sliced
   apples, drained
450g self-raising flour
1 tsp salt
3 tsp ground ginger
3 tsp baking powder
1 tsp bicarbonate soda
225g demerara sugar
175g butter
175g black treacle
175g golden syrup
300ml milk
1 egg, beaten

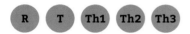

Preheat oven to 170°C. Sift the dry ingredients into a bowl. Heat the butter with the treacle and syrup until melted, allow to cool and then add the milk and egg.

Mix butter/syrup mixture into the dry ingredients.

Line a greased, 23cm square baking tray with baking paper. Place the drained slices of apples neatly in base of the tin. Pour the batter on top of the apples in the tray and bake for 40 minutes.

Test the gingerbread with a skewer to see if it comes out clean. Remove from oven and allow to cool on a wire rack.

Tips: ~Can be served, topped with butter/margarine. ~This dish can be sliced and individually wrapped and frozen for later. Use the ginger bread to make a great dessert—serve with grilled apples and ice cream or with a caramel sauce. ~For a decadent treat, butter the ginger bread slice and pan fry in a non-stick pan, then serve with grilled banana, cream and maple syrup.

Pikelets, jam and cream

Serves 2-3 (makes 8 pikelets) • **Prep** 10 mins • **Cook** 10 mins

1 cup self-raising flour
1 tbsp caster sugar
1¼ cup milk
1 egg
1 tbsp melted butter
Pinch of salt
1 jar of top quality
   seedless jam
3–4 tbsp dollop cream

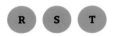

In a mixing bowl, sieve the flour and add the sugar and a pinch of salt. Whisk the milk and eggs together until smooth, add to the dry ingredients, mix well and allow to rest.

Heat a non-stick frypan over medium heat and brush with a little melted butter. Drop 2 level tablespoons full of the mixture into the pan and cook for 30 seconds or until bubbles appear on the surface. Turnover and cook other side for 1 minute, or until golden. Remove and allow to cool.

Spread pikelets with seedless jam and dollop each one with generous helping of cream. Seedless jam can be made by heating a jar of your favourite jam until it melts, passing it through a fine sieve using the back of a kitchen spoon, leaving behind any seeds. Transfer to a scrupulously clean jar and leave sealed in refrigerator once cooled.

Tips: ~These keep well in a sealed airtight container for overnight. ~Clotted cream is a great alternative to serve with the pikelets and can be found in most gourmet food retail outlets. ~They are a quick and ideal mid meal treat and are perfect as part of a high tea component. ~Pikelets can be used as part of a dessert—make them larger and serve with bananas and maple syrup or with ricotta, honey and soft fruits. ~Serve with a drizzle of maple syrup or a blob of the seedless jam and whipped cream.

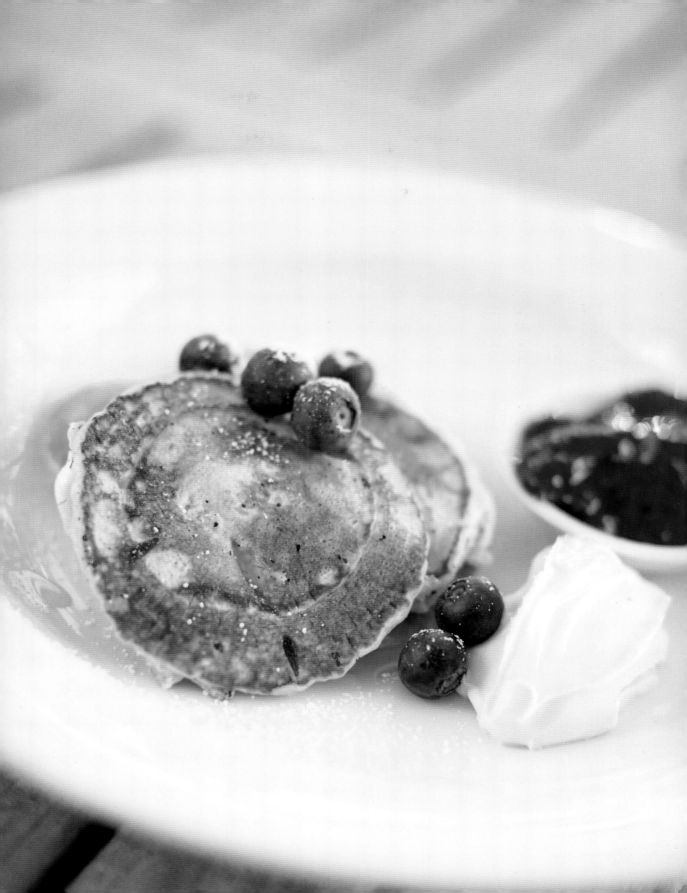

Scones

Serves makes about 6 scones • **Prep** 10 mins • **Cook** 15-20 mins

250g self-raising flour
¼ tsp mixed spice
1 tsp baking powder
5 tbsp (75g) unsalted butter, soft
1½ tbsp (20g) caster sugar
Pinch of salt
150ml milk
Whipped cream and seedless jam to serve

Preheat oven to 190°C, grease a baking tray and line with baking paper. Sift flour, mixed spice, baking powder and salt into a mixing bowl, then add the butter and sugar and rub together until crumbs are formed. Make a well in the crumbs and slowly add most of the milk until it forms a dough with a fork.

Remove and dust a table top with flour, place the dough on the table top and carefully roll to 3 cm height (do not overwork the dough). Add more milk if dry. Cut out into rounds using a cutter. Brush the tops with a little beaten egg and cook in the oven on the middle shelf for 15 minutes.

To check that the scone is ready, turn it over and tap on the bottom—if it is ready, the scone will have a hollow sound. Serve with whipped cream and seedless jam (see method for seedless jam in pikelets recipe).

Tips: ~For a soft diet, minced and moist and smooth pureed diet, follow recipe for soaking foods in Chapter 4. ~Extra scones can be wrapped individually and frozen for eating later.

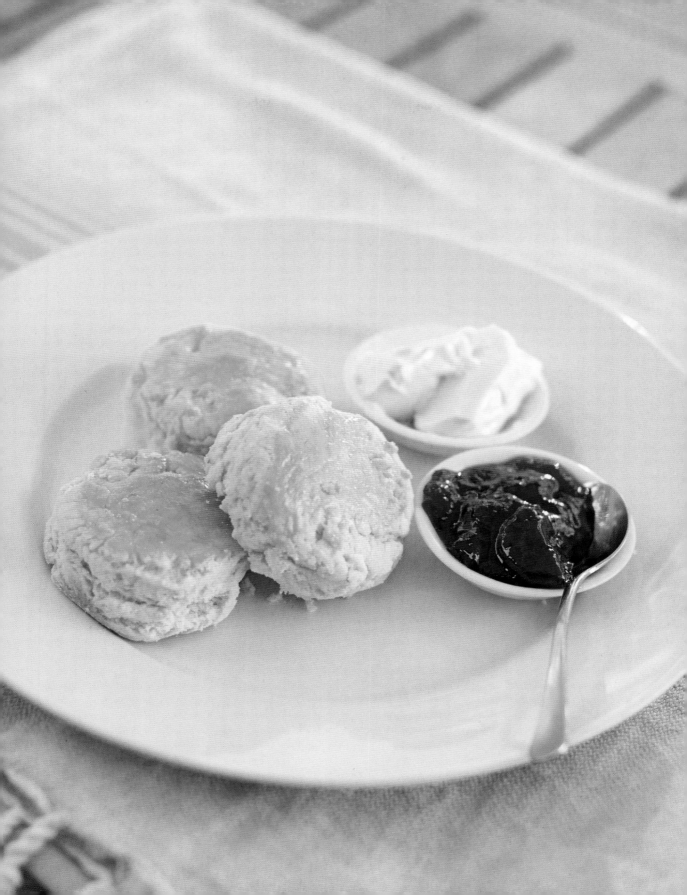

Banana loaf cake

Serves 8 • **Prep** 45 mins • **Cook** 60 mins

2½ cups almond meal
⅔ cups self raising flour
⅔ cups caster sugar
2 tsp cinnamon powder
1 pinch salt
3 very ripe bananas, mashed
2 eggs, beaten
⅔ cups rice bran oil

Topping
2 tbsp demerara sugar
2 tbsp Shredded coconut

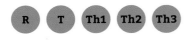

Preheat oven to 180°C. Combine dry ingredients in a mixing well.

In a small bowl, combine the mashed banana, beaten eggs, rice bran oil and baking soda, mix well. Make a well in the centre of the dry ingredients and add the banana and egg mixture. Combine carefully with a wooden spoon (do not over mix).

Grease and line a loaf tin with baking paper and pour the mixture into it. Sprinkle coconut and sugar on top. Bake in the oven for about 60 minutes or until a skewer comes out clean.

Tips: ~Can be kept in the refrigerator for up to 3–4 days. ~Banana loaf slices actually become more moist and taste better after 1 day of refrigeration. ~Batter could also be used for muffins.

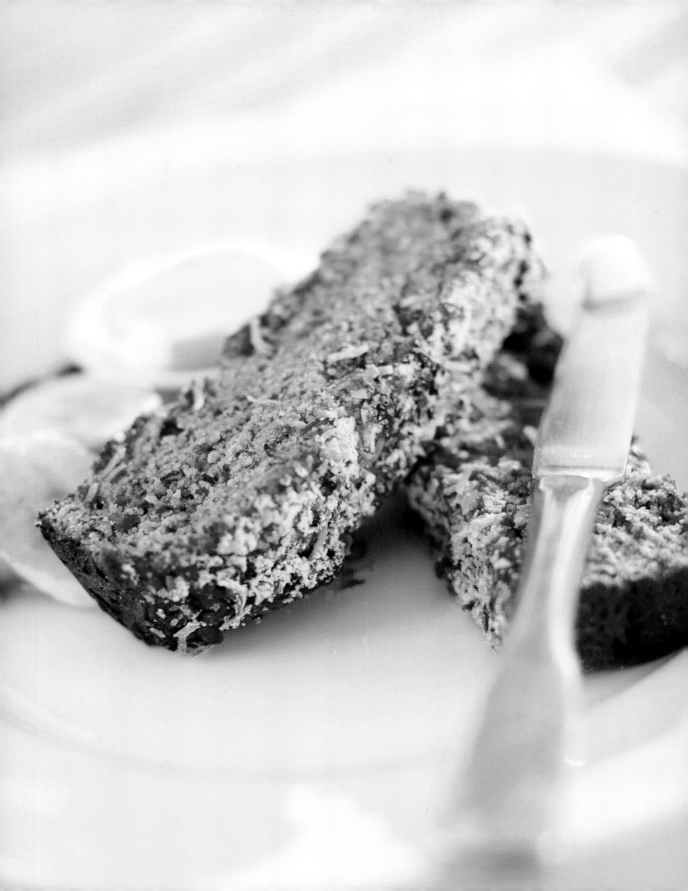

Chocolate semolina 'fudge'

Serves 2-3 • **Prep** 10 mins

1 cup full cream milk
30g (2 tbsp) caster sugar
50g good quality
   dark chocolate
¼ tsp cinnamon
1 tsp vanilla essence
60g fine semolina
   butter for greasing

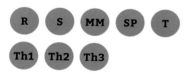

Place milk, sugar and vanilla essence in a saucepan and bring to boil, then add the chocolate and stir to dissolve. Slowly add the semolina and cook for about 3 minutes, stir continuously.

Grease a small square baking tray and carefully pour the chocolate semolina into the tray. You may need to spread the mixture out with the back of a spoon to cover the whole base of the tray. Allow to cool for 1½ hours.

Remove the semolina from the tray (place a plate on top of the semolina and tip the tray upside down) and cut into about 12 slices. Serve on its own as a mid meal or with custard and fruit as a dessert. (One serve is 4-6 pieces).

Tips: ~Ideal finger food or for people on a texture-modified diet. ~Keep refrigerated in a container once cut into pieces. ~People on a puree diet should consume by taking small bites, rather than placing the whole slice in their mouth at once.

Carrot, sultana and walnut cupcakes

Serves makes 8 cupcakes • **Prep** 12 mins • **Cook** 20 mins

1½ cups almond meal
1 tsp cinnamon
1 tsp ground ginger
2 tbsp sultanas
½ tsp baking soda
3 eggs
2 tbsp butter
1½ cups carrot,
    peeled and grated
½ cup walnuts, finely
    chopped
¼ cup honey

Coconut icing
400ml coconut milk
    (leave unopened can in
    refrigerator overnight)
2 tsp maple syrup or honey
1 tsp vanilla extract

Preheat the oven to 180°C. Add the almond meal, cinnamon, ginger, baking soda, sultanas, grated carrot and walnuts in a bowl. Melt the butter and add the honey and stir thoroughly, then add the eggs and beat lightly. Add the butter/egg mixture to the dry ingredients and stir to combine.

Spray 8 cupcake paper cups lightly with olive oil spray and place them in a cupcake tray, pour mixture into the cupcakes papers to the top (this mix does not rise). Sprinkle with the cinnamon and bake for 20 minutes.

Coconut icing
Remove the coconut milk can that has been in the refrigerator overnight, turn upside down and open the can. Carefully scoop out the thickened cream (separates from the milk when refrigerated) into a bowl. To the cream, add the maple syrup and vanilla essence and with a stick blender whip until it resembles whipped cream. Remove the cupcakes from the oven and allow to cool. Spoon on the whipped coconut cream and serve.

Banana and raspberry muffins

Serves makes 6 muffins • **Prep** 10 mins • **Cook** 25 mins

2 cups almond meal
1 cup self-raising flour
⅔ cup soft brown sugar
1 pinch salt
½ cup extra virgin olive oil
2 eggs
2 ripe bananas, mashed
1 tsp vanilla essence
1 tsp cinnamon
¾ cup frozen raspberries

Topping (optional)
1 tbsp demerera sugar
1 tbsp shredded coconut
   for topping

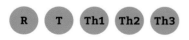

Preheat the oven to 180°C. In a mixing bowl, add the almond meal, sifted self-raising flour, brown sugar, salt and cinnamon together. Make a well in the centre of the mix. In a small bowl, whisk the eggs and add the vanilla essence and olive oil. Carefully mix the wet ingredients with the dry ingredients and add the mashed banana and when all mixed, carefully fold in the frozen raspberries.

Spray 6 large muffin tins with olive oil spray and spoon the muffin mix into all the muffin indentations. Sprinkle demerera sugar and shredded coconut on top (optional) and bake for about 25 minutes, or until a skewer inserted in the muffin comes out clean. Sprinkle with icing sugar and serve.

Tips: ~Other berries can be added instead of the raspberries. ~These muffins freeze well if wrapped and frozen individually. ~They are high in fibre. ~Gluten free self-raising flour can be used.

Vanilla and yoghurt everlasting ice cream

Serves 1 • **Prep** 2 mins • **Cook** 3 mins

100ml vanilla bean
    ice cream
50ml full cream milk
50ml vanilla yoghurt
½ tsp vanilla essence
8 small scoops Spuma
    Instant

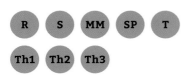

Place all ingredients into a small bowl and stir to combine. Carefully pour into a cream whipper, screw down the top and charge with the cream whipper charger. Shake for 1 minute and place in the refrigerator to cool.

Tips: ~Ideal for any diet. ~A fun way to serve is in ice cream cones (people on a smooth pureed diet are advised not to eat the cones). ~Or just serve in a bowl.

Fruit salad with vanilla honey yoghurt

Prep 2 mins • **Cook** 10 mins

1 cup plain yoghurt
1 tbsp honey
¼ tsp vanilla extract
Juice from ¼ orange
1 tsp of fresh lemon juice
100g strawberries, hulled
    and cut in half
50g blueberries
80g fresh or frozen
    raspberries
1 banana, sliced
100g seedless black grapes

Combine the honey, yoghurt and vanilla and set aside in refrigerator. Into a mixing bowl, slice the banana, then add the lemon juice and the orange juice. Hull and slice the strawberries and add to the banana.

Carefully add the washed grapes, blueberries and finally the fresh raspberries (if using frozen, add them on top of the yoghurt). Place fruit salad into two attractive glasses, top with a generous dollop of the honey vanilla yoghurt and raspberries.

Tips: ~This can be adapted using fruit that is in season and is easy to eat. ~This is perfect as a dessert for lunch, a mid meal snack or for a healthy breakfast. ~If using frozen berries, defrost them overnight on absorbent paper in the fridge.

Raw fruit pudding, coconut icing

Serves 6 • **Prep** 20 mins

80g pitted prunes
1 tsp orange zest
250g pitted dates
80g fine almond meal
2 tbsp sultanas
100g dried apricots
1 tsp grated ginger (fresh)
1 tsp brandy (optional)
1 tsp cinnamon
½ tsp nutmeg
¼ tsp all spice
¼ cup fresh squeezed
   orange juice
1 tbsp butter or coconut oil

Coconut icing
1 can coconut milk
   (refrigerate overnight)
2 tsp maple syrup
1 tsp vanilla extract

Combine all ingredients in a food processor except for the coconut oil and the orange juice. Blend until a smooth crumb-like consistency is reached. Then add the juice and butter/coconut oil, brandy and mix together by hand. Line 6 small dariole moulds or ramekins with plastic wrap and then divide the pudding mix to each mould and pack firmly, then refrigerate for 20 minutes.

Coconut icing
Remove the coconut milk can that has been in the refrigerator overnight, turn upside down and open the can. Carefully scoop out the thickened cream (separates from the milk when refrigerated). The remainder of the milk can be retained for other cooking.

Add the maple syrup and the vanilla extract to the coconut cream and with a stick blender, whip until it thickens to a whipped cream consistency. Remove the puddings from the film and top with the coconut icing.

Tips: ~The pudding mix can be rolled into balls and served as finger food treats (roll in desiccated coconut). ~It can also be heated and served with warm custard for a person on a soft diet. ~It would not need the icing if served with custard. ~The pudding will keep for 3 days if stored in an airtight container in the refrigerator. ~It can be also frozen.

Tomato jelly, basil and goat's curd

Serves 1 • **Prep** 5 mins • **Cook** 15 mins

Tomato jelly
(makes about 400ml
= 2 serves)

750g ripe tomatoes
1 clove garlic
¼ Spanish onion,
    finely sliced
½ cup picked basil leaves
4 small scoops Gelea Instant
Basil pesto (makes 4 serves)
20 basil leaves
1 tsp shaved parmesan
1 tsp almond meal
2 tbsp extra virgin olive oil
½ clove garlic

To finish
Goat's curd or ricotta cheese
    (2 tbsp per serve)

Tips: ~This recipe should make about 400ml of tomato stock but you will only need 200ml for the jelly. ~Any leftover stock can be frozen and used another time.

Wash and remove stems from tomatoes and chop into a large rough dice. Place onion, garlic, tomato and basil into a food processor or blender. Blend the tomato until it resembles a thick soup-like consistency (it may require two batches to blend all the pulp).

Place the mixture into a stainless steel saucepan and bring to a simmer. Do not allow to boil rapidly. Carefully remove some of the scum from the surface. Allow to cool slightly. Pass the clear tomato stock through a fine sieve, discarding any sediment or scum left in the sieve.

Place 200mls of the tomato stock into a small stainless steel saucepan, add the Gelea Instant to the stock and stir. Bring the stock to a simmer and stir constantly for 3 minutes. Remove from heat and allow to cool slightly, then pour into a glass or small china bowl and refrigerate until cold and set.

To make the pesto
Place all pesto ingredients in a small food processor and blend until a smooth paste. Alternatively place in a cup and use a stick blender to turn into a paste, add a little more oil if it is too dry. Ensure there are no lumps in the pesto. For a smooth pureed diet or a thickened fluid diet, ensure that all oil is removed from the pesto, or thicken the pesto with a commercial thickener (to desired consistency).

To finish the dish
Place a generous spoonful of pesto on the chilled tomato jelly. In a small stainless steel bowl place 2 tbsp of goat's curd and mix with a teaspoon just to soften slightly, scoop and place on top of the pesto.

Pete's arancini

Serves 4-6 • **Prep** 30 mins • **Cook** 20 mins

160g Arborio rice
160ml milk
160ml water
35g butter

Filling
60g ham, finely diced
60g mozzarella cheese,
grated
80g eggplant, finely diced
1 tbsp olive oil
60g parmesan cheese,
   grated
1g (pinch) sea salt
Pepper to taste

For the panade
(breadcrumbing)
1 small bowl sifted flour
1 small bowl with 1 egg and
50ml milk whisked together
   and seasoned (egg wash)
1 small bowl of fine
   breadcrumbs

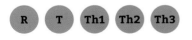

Add the milk, water and butter to a small stainless steel saucepan, bring to the boil, then add the rice and and simmer with lid on until the rice is cooked, stir only once or twice. Remove from heat.

Skin, finely dice and then fry the eggplant in the olive oil until soft and lightly golden. Add the remainder of the filling ingredients to the eggplant, then add the rice mix and stir until combined. Season to taste, then allow to cool.

With slightly wet, clean hands mould the rice mixture into balls—should make 6 x 125g balls (these can be made smaller for finger food). With clean hands, coat the balls in the flour, then the egg wash and for the final stage, toss the balls with the breadcrumbs.

The arancini balls can then be sprayed with a little oil and baked in a preheated oven until golden brown.

Tips: ~These freeze well and are ideal for finger food or lunch with a salad. ~They are also great served with the 'Tomato sauce' recipe. ~High in protein.

Cheese and tomato custards

Serves 2 • **Prep** 10 mins • **Cook** 20 mins

60g grated mozzarella
  cheese
1 tbsp parmesan cheese
1 cup milk
1 egg, beaten lightly
1/2 tsp Dijon mustard
a pinch of cayenne pepper
  (to taste)
Salt and pepper
3 tsp tomato paste

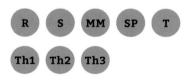

Preheat oven to 130°C. Stir the milk and the cheeses over a low heat until melted (do not boil), remove from the heat and allow to cool. Add the egg and mustard and season with salt and pepper and a pinch of cayenne pepper.

Grease (with butter) 2 small ramekins and spoon the tomato paste in the bottom of each ramekin and smear over the base. Strain the cheese mix through a sieve and pour carefully into the 2 ramekins. Cover the ramekins with baking paper and foil to inhibit a crust forming.

Place in oven and bake for 20 minutes or until the centre of the custard starts to set. Allow to cool slightly and firm up before serving.

Tips: This is a great savoury treat, high in protein and calcium.

Welsh rare-bit

Serves 1 • **Prep** 10 mins • **Cook** 10 mins

70g cheddar cheese,
   grated coarsely
1 tsp Dijon mustard
15g butter
1 tbsp Guinness
1 dash Worcestershire sauce
1 slice of toasted sourdough
   bread with butter on
   one side
Pinch of sea salt
Two pinches of pepper

(R) (T)

Place butter in a saucepan and melt it. Add the Guinness, a pinch of salt and a couple of pinches of pepper. When close to boiling add the cheese, mustard and the dash of Worcestershire sauce, stirring lightly to help melt the cheese. Do not let it boil.

Place the cheese mixture on top of the buttered side of the sourdough. Place under the grill until browned slightly.

Tips: ~Caution, the cheese will be very hot, so eat with a knife and fork—this is not a finger food. ~High in energy and protein. ~Don't forget to finish off the rest of the Guinness!

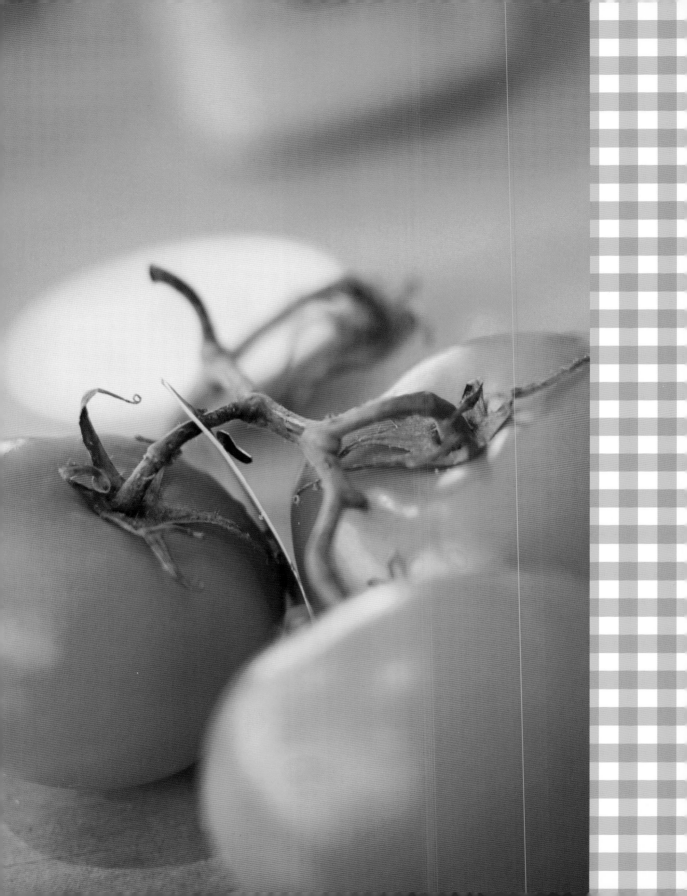

Lunch

Whether you are busy and looking for quick but tasty options, or it's a chance to pause and share the joy of favourite foods, our lunch recipes will hit the spot on a cold winter's day or warm summer afternoon.

Bacon and lentil soup with crusty sourdough bread

Serves 3 • **Prep** 5 mins • **Cook** 50 mins

1 tbsp olive oil
1 onion, finely diced
1 stalk of celery, diced
1 carrot, peeled and diced
2 cloves garlic, finely
    chopped
1 tsp cumin
90g French green lentils,
    washed and checked for
    stones
3 rashers of lean bacon, rind
    removed and diced
900ml chicken stock
½ can (200g) diced tomatoes
¼ savoy cabbage, finely
    shredded
Salt and pepper to taste
1 tbsp parsley, chopped
    (to serve)
2 tbsp sour cream (to serve)
3 x crusty sourdough
    bread rolls

Place half the olive oil in a heavy-based saucepan.
Fry the bacon until it is brown and drain any excess fat.
Remove bacon from pan and allow to continue draining on absorbent paper. Place the rest of the olive oil in the pan, add the onion and stir until translucent (but not browned).

Add the garlic, carrot, celery, washed lentils, cumin, stock and canned tomatoes. Stir together. Bring to boil, then reduce heat and simmer for 40 minutes. Skim the surface with a slotted spoon to remove any scum.

Add the cabbage and season the soup with salt and cracked black pepper. Return the bacon to the saucepan and stir. Serve to 3 bowls with a dollop of sour cream and a sprinkle of the parsley. Serve with crusty sourdough bread rolls.

Tips: ~This soup can be spiced up with fresh diced chilli, perfect for a rainy winter day.
~If you are not able to find French green lentils, you can use any type of lentil.

Reuben sandwich
with sauerkraut

Serves 2 • **Prep** 5 mins

4 thick slices of white,
   wholemeal or rye bread
150g sauerkraut (canned),
   squeezed dry and drained
   of any moisture
120g Gruyere cheese, sliced
150g sliced pastrami
20g chopped cornichons
   or small gherkins
1 tbsp parsley, chopped
½ tbsp Dijon mustard
1-2 tbsp Thousand Island
   dressing
1 tsp softened butter
Salt and pepper to taste

Lightly butter one side of all four sides of the bread, smear other sides with a little Dijon mustard. Place 2 slices of the bread buttered-side down and divide the pastrami onto both slices of bread (this should be the mustard side).

Mix the sauerkraut with the chopped parsley, chopped cornichons and enough Thousand Island dressing to moisten the sauerkraut slightly. Divide sauerkraut mixture equally onto the pastrami. Place the Gruyere cheese equally on top of the sauerkraut. Place the two remaining bread slices on top to complete the sandwiches (buttered-side should be on the outside of the sandwiches).

These can be cooked in a sandwich maker or in a hot frying pan until golden on both sides. If using the frying pan, be careful the sandwiches do not burn.

Tips: ~Cut the sandwiches in half and serve with a green salad and potato salad. ~Corned beef can be used rather than pastrami. ~When making a sandwich always season each layer with salt and pepper. ~This dish is a good source of protein, calcium iron and fibre (especially when using rye bread).

Mushroom and ham frittata

Serves 2 • **Prep** 10 mins • **Cook** 15 mins

4 eggs
3 tsp butter
¼ cup cream
1 tbsp flat leaf parsley,
    chopped
1 cup field mushrooms,
    sliced
120g leg ham, diced
100g mozzarella cheese,
    grated
Salt and pepper to taste
Green salad and crusty
    bread to serve

In a bowl, whisk together eggs, cream, salt, pepper and parsley, then set aside. Melt 1 teaspoon of the butter in an ovenproof, non-stick pan over a medium heat. Add mushrooms and ham and cook, stirring occasionally until mushrooms are just tender (about 4–5 minutes). Add the mushroom-ham mixture to the egg mixture in the bowl, stirring constantly.

Melt the remaining butter into the same small ovenproof, non-stick pan. Add egg mixture and cook, stirring occasionally and running a heatproof rubber spatula around the edges from time to time, until eggs are just set and bottom is golden brown (about 3–4 minutes).

Sprinkle cheese on top of the frittata and transfer to oven. Cook until eggs are completely set and cheese is golden brown (about 2–3 minutes). Serve with garden salad and sliced crusty bread with butter.

Tips: ~Any combination can be added to this process, such as tomato, chicken, or make it a vegetarian option (just omit the ham). ~You can make finger food sized frittatas by pouring the egg mixture into small, greased muffin tins (the recipe should make about 4 patties).

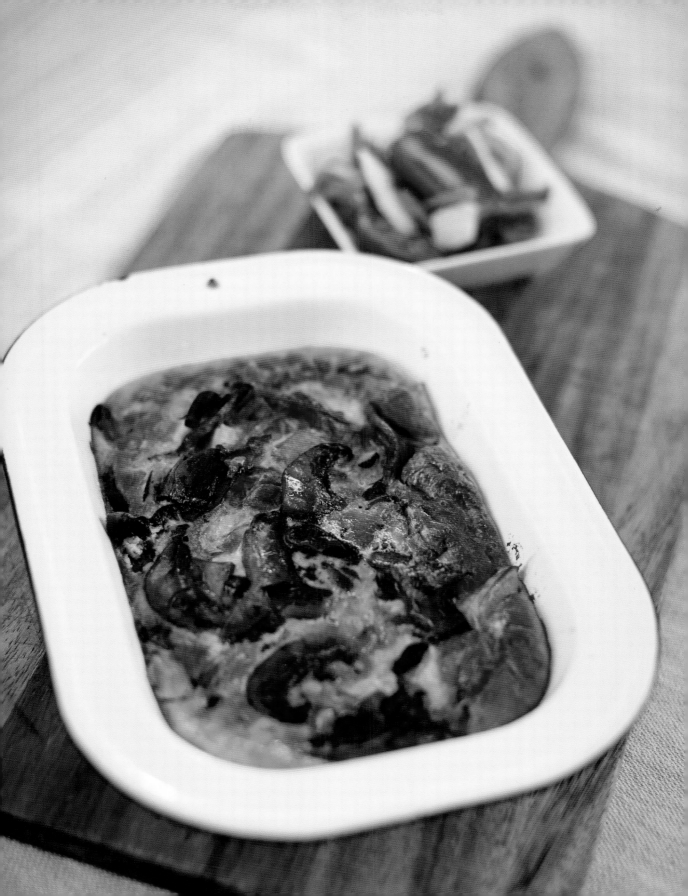

Pea and salmon fishcakes with tartare sauce

Serves 2 • **Prep** 10 mins • **Cook** 10 mins

Fishcake
50g frozen peas
150g salmon fillet, skin off
150g potato, peeled
   and diced
½ tbsp parsley, chopped
½ lemon, zested and juiced
1 egg
1 tbsp plain flour
Salt and pepper to taste
1 pinch of nutmeg

Fishcake crumb coating
100g plain flour
1 egg, beaten
100g fine breadcrumbs or
   4 slices crustless bread,
   blend in food processor
2 tbsp olive oil

Toppings
Tartare sauce
(See 'Basic recipes')

Put a saucepan of water on to boil and add salt. Once boiling, blanch the peas for 20 seconds. Drain under cold running water and place in a bowl. Place potatoes in salted water and bring to boil. Cook until potatoes are soft.

Rub salmon fillet with olive oil and season with salt and pepper. Place salmon on top of the cooking potatoes in a colander or sieve to steam. Cover with foil. When potatoes and salmon are both cooked remove and allow to cool.

Place the peas Into a mixing bowl, then flake the salmon on top and crumble the potatoes. Season well with salt and pepper, add the zest and juice of the lemon, the beaten egg, and the finely sliced green shallots and parsley. Mix together, then add the plain flour and pinch of nutmeg.

Make 4 patties out of the fishcake mix. Crumb each patty– put the flour, eggs and breadcrumbs into three separate bowls. Put each patty first through the flour, then the egg and finally the breadcrumbs. Leave in thefridge until you are ready to cook them.

When you are ready to eat, preheat the oven to 180°C. Pour the olive oil into a frying pan with a small knob of butter and turn the heat to medium. Lay the fishcakes in the pan and cook for about 2–3 minutes until they are brown on both sides. Remove the partly cooked fishcakes from the pan and finish cooking in the oven for 7 minutes on an ovenproof tray.

Serve fishcakes with tartare sauce. Accompany the fishcakes with a hearty salad, even some hot chips.

Tips: ~Salmon fillet can be substituted with canned salmon. ~Drain the excess liquid and pick out the bones.

Homemade pizza

Serves 4 • **Prep** 30 mins (plus about 1 hour for dough to prove) • **Cook** 10—15 mins

Making the pizza dough
350g strong (baker's) flour,
plus extra to dust work
surface
1 tsp caster sugar
1 x 7g packet dried
   instant yeast
2 tbsp olive oil
2 tsp salt
250ml warm water

Pizza topping
2 x 140g pizza sauce
150g buffalo mozzarella
Extra virgin olive oil,
   to drizzle
30g Parmesan cheese,
   grated
6 slices (100g) prosciutto or
   ham, torn into pieces
10 cherry tomatoes, halved
¼ bunch washed basil
   leaves, picked and torn
Pepper to taste

Rocket Salad
2 cups rocket leaves, washed
50g shaved Parmesan
   cheese
2 tbsp olive oil
1 tsp balsamic dressing

Preheat the oven to 200°C. Measure out 1 cup (250ml) warm water into a jug. Add 1 tablespoon of the flour to a bowl. Add the caster sugar, yeast and 3 tablespoons of the warm water.

Stir briefly to combine, then let stand in a warm place for 10 minutes or until large bubbles appear on the surface. Sift the remaining flour into a large bowl. Add the yeast mixture, olive oil, remaining warm water and 2 teaspoons salt. Bring the mixture together with your hands, then turn onto a lightly floured surface. Knead for at least 5 minutes or until the dough is smooth.

Rub a new bowl with oil. Place the ball of dough in it, then cover with a damp tea towel and set aside in a warm draft free place to prove (rise) for about 1 hour or until dough has doubled in size. Lightly grease two 26cm pizza trays and dust with a little flour, or cover with baking paper.

Turn the dough out onto a floured surface. Knock the air out of the dough by punching it with your fist, then divide into 2 pieces and knead each one into a smooth ball. Dust a rolling pin with flour and roll out the dough into rounds about 20cm in diameter. Lay onto the prepared pizza trays, then use your hands to press the dough out slightly and spread the bases liberally with pizza sauce.

Slice the buffalo mozzarella, then pat dry with absorbent paper to absorb any excess moisture. Drizzle the pizza bases with a little olive oil, and then arrange mozzarella and Parmesan on top, followed by the torn prosciutto/ham and cherry tomato halves.

recipe continues...

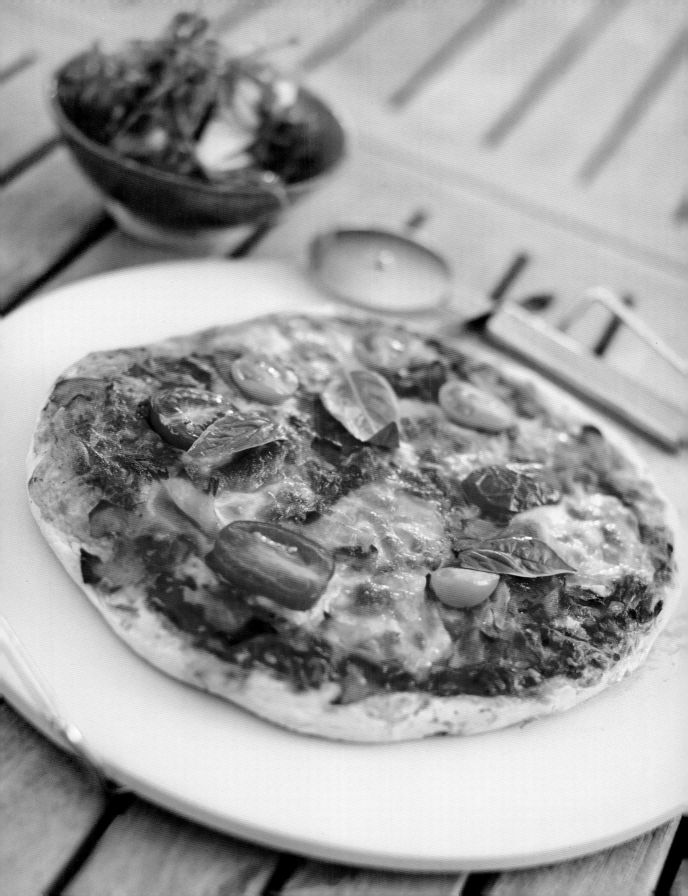

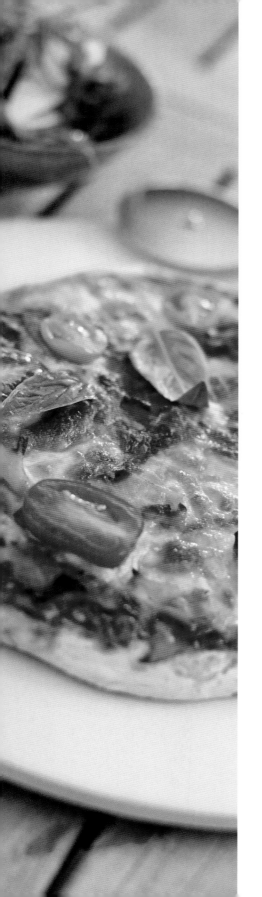

Homemade pizza

Place pizzas in the oven and bake for 5–7 minutes, or until the bases are crisp, golden and the cheese has melted. Remove from the oven and top pizzas with torn basil leaves (they will wilt slightly). Sprinkle with freshly ground black pepper and drizzle with a little more olive oil. Slice and serve immediately.

Making the rocket salad
Add the washed rocket, Parmesan, olive oil and balsamic vinegar to a bowl and toss. Serve with the pizza.

Tips: ~While this recipe includes a homemade pizza dough, you can purchase pre-made bases from the supermarket (either fresh or frozen). ~You can also use a flatbread, such as pita or tortilla, as a base. ~These can all be kept in the freezer. ~Pizza is great for using leftovers or making a favourite combination for each member of the family. You can make any combination of vegetarian pizza– simply omit the prosciutto/ham and replace with another type of protein. ~Thicker bases are better for finger food, as they hold their shape better. ~You can preserve leftover basil by chopping and freezing in just enough oil or water to cover. ~Use an ice-cube tray for portions that can be added to soups, casseroles or stir-fries. ~Pizza slices can be frozen raw and then cooked. ~Cooked slices can be stored in the fridge and microwaved the next day.

Hearty ploughman's lunch

Serves 2 • **Prep** 10 mins

1 egg boiled, halved
60g leg ham sliced
2 x 30g wedges aged
cheddar cheese
25 g mustard pickles
    or piccalilli
4 gherkins
4 pickled onions
1 stick of celery, thinly sliced
½ cup beetroot, sliced and
    drained (optional)
Leaf salad mix (100g)
8 cherry tomatoes, or one
    tomato cut into wedges
¼ cucumber, sliced
2 tbsp Olive oil
1 tbsp white wine vinegar
4 slices crusty bread
Butter or margarine, at
    room-temperature

Make the dressing by adding white wine vinegar and olive oil together and stir to combine. In a bowl, dress the salad leaves with the dressing. Arrange other ingredients on a share plate or onto two plates. Serve immediately.

Tips: ~This style of meal is ideal for grazing and snacking over lunch. ~Fingers or forks are both suitable. ~It's a really easy lunch, ideal for summer |and easily served on a tray for a picnic. ~Any combination is good! ~Use whatever you have in the fridge—the secret to this meal is a nice presentation! ~You can add a slice of quiche or slice of pork pie or add Spanish onion, tomato and cucumber to the salad. ~To make more salad dressing, you can use this easy formula—1 part vinegar to 2 parts olive oil.

R T

Meatloaf with simple tomato chutney

Serves 4 • **Prep** 20 mins • **Cook** 40 mins

For the Meatloaf
500g extra lean beef mince
1 cup fresh wholemeal
    breadcrumbs
1 small brown onion, grated
    or very finely diced (no
    more than 0.5cm pieces)
1 carrot, peeled and
    coarsely grated
1 celery stick, finely chopped
2 tbsp tomato sauce
2 tbsp flat-leaf parsley
    leaves, chopped
1 egg, lightly beaten
1 tsp Dijon mustard
1 tsp salt
¾ tsp cracked black pepper
2 tsp Worcestershire sauce

*Tomato chutney–see
'Basic recipes'*

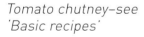
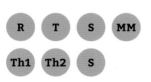

Preheat oven to 180°C. Line a baking tray or loaf tin with baking paper. Place mince, breadcrumbs, onion, carrot, celery, tomato sauce, Worcestershire sauce, Dijon mustard, parsley and egg in a large bowl. Season with salt and pepper. Using clean hands, mix until well combined.

Press mince into tin or shape into a rectangle and place on the prepared baking tray. Bake for 25 to 30 minutes or until firm to touch. Remove from oven and drain any excess fat.

Make the tomato chutney and place in the fridge until ready to serve. Use a commercial thickener to thicken the chutney to appropriate consistency. Slice the meatloaf and serve with steamed vegetables and potatoes, or green salad and a bread roll (omit bread roll for minced and moist diet. For a soft diet, serve with soft bread).

Tips: ~This is an easy recipe to make in bulk and freeze. ~Place baking paper or cling wrap between portions. ~You can process the chutney with a hand mixer or put through a mouli for a smoother relish.

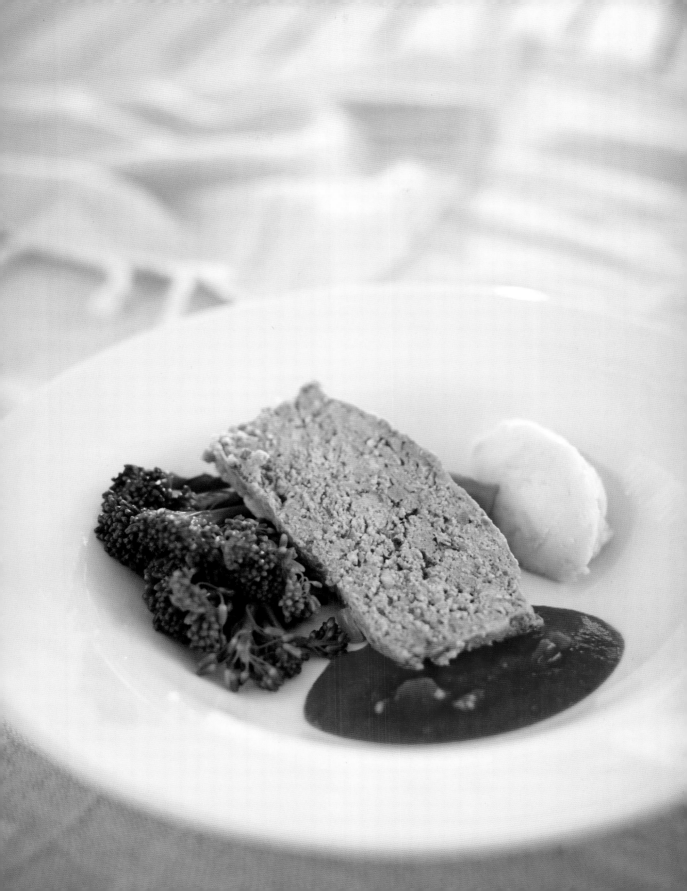

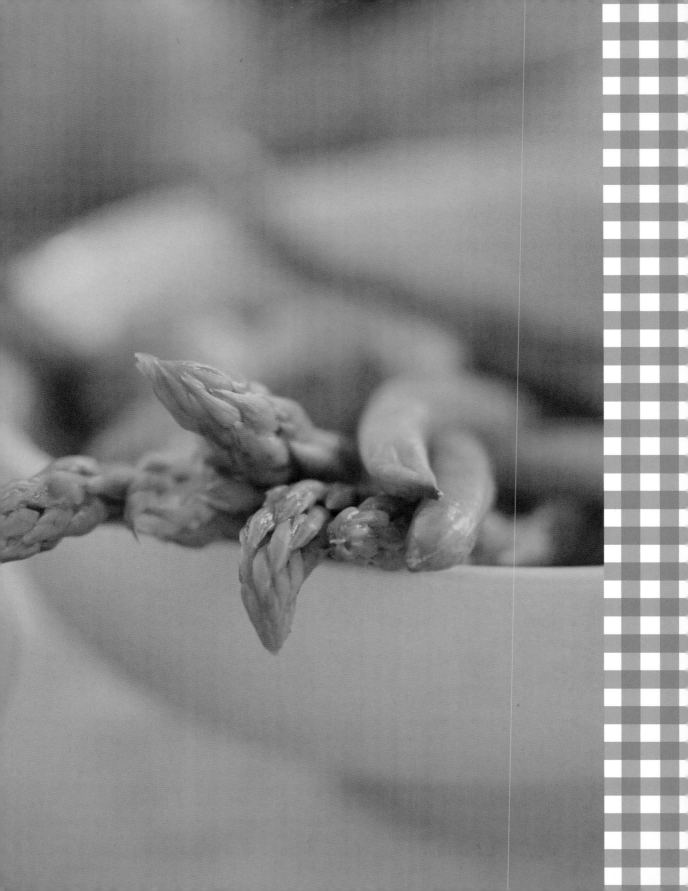

Dinner

Dinner can be an opportunity for older people to reflect on the day, or on lifetime memories, as well as to catch up with family and friends. We've created a multicultural range of recipes suitable for an intimate dinner for two or a big family celebration while at the same time meeting the dietary needs of older people and people living with dementia.

Semolina gnocchi
with tomato and olive stew

Serves 2 • **Prep** 15 mins • **Cook** 25 mins

For the gnocchi
450ml milk
120g semolina
50g Parmesan cheese, grated
¾ tsp pepper
Pinch of nutmeg
4 basil leaves
1 tsp salt
1 egg yolk
20g butter
1 sprig of rosemary
2 bay leaves

For the Tomato stew
½ Spanish onion,
    cut into 6 wedges
2 cloves garlic, thinly sliced
60g or 6 small cherry
    tomatoes
1 vine ripened tomato,
    blanched, skin and seeds
    removed
½ punnet yellow teardrop
    tomatoes or other
    heirloom small tomatoes
10 Ligurian olives, seeded
    and split into two
75ml olive oil
¼ tsp fresh thyme leaves,
    chopped
½ tsp sage leaves, chopped
Salt and pepper to taste
8–10 basil leaves
    (for garnishing)

Preheat oven to 200°C. In a saucepan, add the milk, nutmeg, rosemary, basil, bay leaves and salt and pepper and bring to the boil. Remove the bay leaves, basil leaves and rosemary. Gradually add in the semolina, while whisking. Whisk until smooth and cook for 3 minutes. Remove from heat, then add butter, egg yolk, Parmesan cheese and beat the mixture well with a wooden spoon.

Grease a non-stick surface or container with olive oil. Spoon out the gnocchi mix into the container or tray and spread with a pastry scraper to make a neat square (about 1cm in thickness). Melt the butter and brush the surface of the gnocchi square. Sprinkle the freshly grated Parmesan on top of the buttered gnocchi square.

For the tomato and olive stew, add a dash of olive oil in a non-stick frying pan. Add the onion 'petals' and cook on a low heat until transparent—do not allow to burn. Add the garlic and then cut the seeded tomatoes halves into petals. Add the 75ml olive oil and all of the yellow teardrop tomatoes and cherry tomatoes into the frying pan. Simmer until tomatoes begin to soften, and then add the olives, sage and thyme. Season with salt and pepper and then remove from the heat.

Cut the gnocchi into 6 rectangular wedges. Place the wedges on baking paper and place them in the oven until golden brown. Carefully remove the gnocchi from the tray. Place 3 rectangles on each plate and put a generous amount of tomato and olive stew next to them. Sprinkle liberally with picked basil leaves. Drizzle with a little extra olive oil.

R T

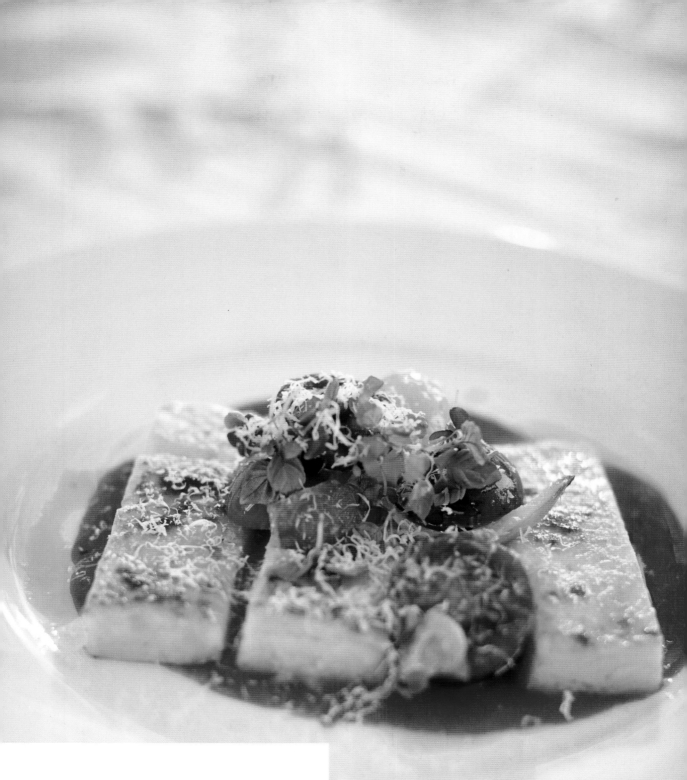

Tip: This is a great vegetarian meal.

Duck sausage with braised lentils

Serves 2 • **Prep** 15 mins • **Cook** 20 mins

Duck Sausage
250g duck Maryland,
    skin off and deboned
1 tbsp pork fat or
    diced duck skin
1 tsp salt
2 tsp olive oil
1 tbsp onions, finely diced
1 clove garlic, finely
    chopped
½ tsp black pepper
½ tsp all spice (nutmeg,
    cinnamon, cloves)
½ tsp fennel seeds, ground
½ tbsp parsley, chopped
¼ tbsp thyme, chopped
½ tsp ground ginger
Zest from ¼ orange
2 tsp chopped pistachio
    nuts
2 cups panko bread
    crumbs (available from
    the supermarket) or
    fresh white breadcrumbs
    (remove crust from sliced
    bread and process in food
    processor until fine).
Butter for cooking

Braised Lentils
1 x 400g tin lentils,
    drained and washed
    (should yield 250g)
25g butter

1 tbsp onion, diced
½ clove garlic, sliced
¼ medium carrot, diced
200ml chicken stock
½ tbsp parsley, chopped
¼ tsp ground coriander
¼ tsp ground fennel
2 cups baby spinach leaves
Salt and pepper to taste

Place duck, fat and all the spices and salt in a food processor. Heat the oil in a pan and gently cook the onion and garlic. Remove from heat and allow to cool. Place the cooled onion and garlic mix (with the oil) in the food processor with all the other ingredients except the pistachio nuts and blend. Finally add the pistachio nuts.

Place the sausage mix in the freezer for 30 mins to firm. Remove from freezer and form into 4 sausages (surplus sausages can be wrapped and frozen for later use). Roll into breadcrumbs.

To prepare the lentils, place butter into a heavy based saucepan. Add the onion and cook gently until translucent. Add the garlic and cook for a minute. Add the carrot and stock, simmer until carrots are cooked. Season with spices, and then add lentils. Simmer for another minute and season with salt and pepper. Spinach leaves can be wilted in the hot lentils and placed on a hot plate.

Heat a knob of butter in a frying pan and cook the sausages. When browned, turn over until all sides are golden. Serve the sausages on the warm lentils.

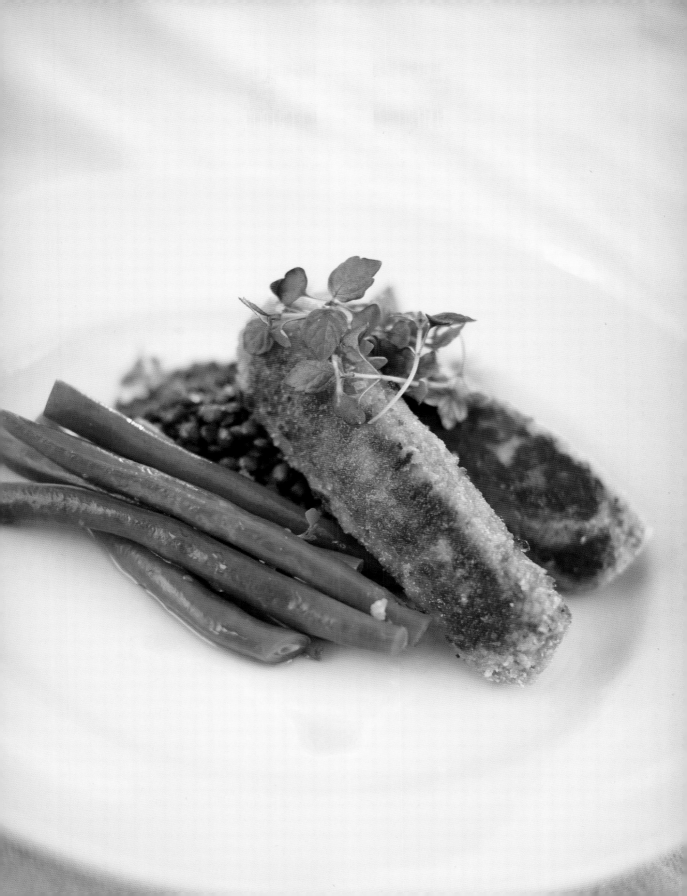

Roast chicken breast, cannellini bean puree, roasted tomatoes

Serves 2 • **Prep** 15 mins • **Cook** 30 mins

1 large (about 220g) breast
   of chicken, skin on
½ punnet (about 125g)
   cherry tomatoes
3 tbsp olive oil
½ can (420g can) cannellini
   beans, drained and
   washed
1 garlic clove
½ brown onion, diced
½ small carrot, diced
2 tbsp celery, finely diced
1 cup chicken stock
1 cup tomato passata
   (thick tomato puree,
   available in supermarket)
25g butter
½ sprig of thyme
Juice from a ¼ lemon
Salt and pepper,
   season to taste

R **T**

Preheat oven to 180°C. Rub the skin of the chicken with a little sea salt. Add 1 tbsp of olive oil and sprinkle with pepper. Heat a little oil in a frying pan, brown the skin of the chicken breast. Turn over to brown the underside also. Throw in the sprig of thyme and add the butter. Allow to melt and carefully squeeze the lemon into the butter mixture. Turn off the heat.

Place the chicken breast on baking paper in a small ovenproof dish. Pour over the pan juices. Add cherry tomatoes to the chicken breast dish, drizzle 1 tbsp of olive oil over both the chicken and the tomatoes and season the tomatoes. Place the chicken and tomatoes in the oven and cook for 15 minutes or until chicken is fully cooked.

Heat a saucepan and brown the onion with a little olive oil, add the garlic, celery and carrot, cooking until it starts to look golden. Add the stock and simmer for 5 minutes, then add the cannellini beans and cook for 10 more minutes.

Drain a little of the stock from the cannellini beans and reserve. Blend the beans and vegetables, adjusting the consistency with a little of the reserved stock until it has the consistency of mashed potato. Then add the rest of the butter and season.

Warm the tomato passata sauce and season. Place a scoop of bean puree on plates, pour the hot tomato passata next to the puree. Cut the chicken in half and place on top of the puree. Place the cherry tomatoes alongside.

Tips: ~The cannellini puree is great with meat or fish, or as a vegetarian dish (just use vegetable stock). ~It's also ideal as a dip—just drizzle olive oil in the puree and serve with crackers or sliced vegetable sticks.

Pan fried ocean trout, potato cake and pea puree

Serves 2 • **Prep** 20 mins • **Cook** 20 mins

Ocean Trout
2 x 120g ocean trout or
    salmon fillet, pin boned
    and skin on
Dash of olive oil
Salt and pepper for
    seasoning

Potato Cake (makes 2 cakes)
350g Maris Piper or
    Desiree potatoes,
    peeled and cut
    into large dices
40ml cream
1 egg yolk
25g Gruyere cheese, grated
40g Parmesan cheese,
    grated
Zest of ½ lemon
1 pinch nutmeg
25g butter
1 garlic clove
¼ onion, chopped
½ tbsp parsley, chopped
Salt and pepper to taste

Pea and herb puree
125 ml chicken stock
250g frozen peas
2 tbsp chopped onion
½ tbsp. butter
1 tsp chopped mint
1 tsp chopped parsley
Salt and pepper for
    seasoning

Potato cake
In a saucepan place potatoes, some salt and top with water. Bring to boil. When cooked, strain off the water. Heat a saucepan with butter and fry the onions. Add the garlic and then add the drained potatoes and cream. Remove from heat and mash the potatoes and season to taste with salt and pepper. Add Parmesan and Gruyere cheese, egg yolk, parsley and nutmeg. Fold through the potato cake mix. Form potato mix into 2 patties and refrigerate for later use.

Pea puree
Bring chicken stock to the boil, add the onion and garlic and simmer for 2 minutes and then add the peas. Bring the peas back to the boil and turn down to simmer until peas are cooked. Strain the liquid, retaining for later. Add the butter to the cooked drained peas and start to blend the peas with a stick blender, adding the retained stock gradually to peas until a firm puree texture is achieved. When consistency is correct add the chopped parsley and mint, taste the puree and add salt and pepper to taste. Keep warm.

Ocean trout
Heat a pan and add a dash of olive oil. Cook the 2 fillets of ocean trout or salmon with the skin side down until the skin is crispy.

At the same time, also cook the potato cakes until they are lightly browned.

Turn the fish over and continue until fish is cooked to your liking. Do the same for the potato cakes. Serve on plates with lemon wedge, pea puree and browned potato cakes.

Tips: ~Any fish fillet can be used for this recipe. ~Chopped ham or cooked diced bacon can be added to the potato cakes. ~A good source of calcium and protein.

Pickled pork neck, red cabbage and mustard sauce

Serves 4-6 • **Prep** 25 mins (complete first step the night before) • **Cook** 1½-2 hrs

Pork neck
750g pickled pork neck
   (pre-order from butcher)
½ onion, peeled and
   cut in half
1 stalk of celery, sliced
1 carrot, peeled and
   chopped in half
½ tsp peppercorns
1 bay leaf
2 cloves of garlic
1 tbsp white wine vinegar
½ tbsp brown sugar

Mustard Sauce
20g butter
¼ onion, finely chopped
½ tbsp plain flour
½ cup beef stock
¼ cup pickling liquid
1 tsp Dijon mustard
¼ cup cream
1 tbsp parsley, coarsely
   chopped

Cabbage
1 tbsp butter
½ onion, thinly sliced
1 Granny Smith apple,
   peeled, cored and thinly
   sliced
400g (about ½ small head)
   red cabbage, cored,
   halved and sliced thinly
1 tbsp sultanas
3 tbsp white wine vinegar
4 tsp brown sugar
½ cup water
Salt and pepper

Serve with
1 kg small chat potatoes or
   Kipfler potatoes
2 tbsp chopped parsley
3 tbsp butter
Salt and pepper to taste

R **T**

Place pork in a large pot and cover with water. Leave overnight in the fridge. The next day, drain the pork and cover with cold water. Bring to boil and skim regularly. Add onion, celery, carrot, peppercorns, bay leaf, garlic, vinegar and brown sugar. Simmer until very tender (about 1½–2 hours). Remove pork neck carefully and insert a skewer—if there is great resistance it may need to be cooked longer.

recipe continues...

Story behind the dish: This is a traditional Welsh recipe I grew up eating. It actually tastes more like ham than pork, due to the neck being pickled. PMJ

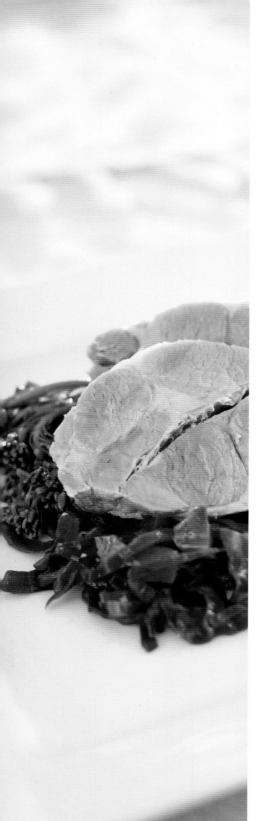

Pickled pork neck, red cabbage and mustard sauce

Place the washed potatoes in a large saucepan of salted cold water and cook for 15–20 mins or until cooked through, drain and season with salt and pepper, then add the butter and keep warm til ready to serve.

To prepare the cabbage, heat the butter in a heavy saucepan, add the onion and cook until translucent. Add the apple and cook for 3 minutes. Add the red cabbage, water and vinegar. Bring to boil and stir until cabbage is cooked (15–20 minutes). Season to taste, then add sultanas and brown sugar.

To make the sauce, melt the butter in a saucepan. Add onion and cook over low heat until soft. Add flour and cook for 1 minute. Gradually add the beef stock and pickling liquid. Cook until mixture thickens. Stir in mustard and cream and simmer for 2 minutes. Add the chopped parsley.

Remove the pork from the hot liquid. Slice and serve with the sauce and red cabbage. Place the warm potatoes in a ceramic bowl and sprinkle with chopped parsley. Place on the table for guests to serve themselves.

Tips: ~Pre-order the pickled pork neck from your local butcher. Ask for it to be tied in netting. ~Left over pork can be used for sandwiches the next day if refrigerated and the cold cabbage (if any leftover) is great accompaniment in the sandwich.

Slow braised beef cheeks with parsnip puree

Serves 3-4 • **Prep** 10 mins • **Cook** 3 hrs

500–600g beef cheeks
40ml olive oil
1 carrot, chopped into a
   large dice
1 stalk of celery, sliced
1 bulb garlic, diced
¼ orange zest
1 brown onion, sliced
300ml red wine (Shiraz)
200ml beef stock
2 bay leaves
1 tbsp thyme leaves
1 tsp salt
1 tsp black pepper
2 cups green vegetables
   to serve, such as peas,
   broccoli or green beans

Parsnip puree
Refer to parsnip puree
in 'Basic recipes'.

Trim the beef cheeks to remove any sinew and silver skin and neaten them up. Season with salt and pepper. Heat half the olive oil in a large heavy-based saucepan over high heat. Brown the beef cheeks for 2 minutes on each side (or until golden), and then remove from the pan. Add the remaining olive oil, and then add the carrot, garlic, onion and celery, cooking over high heat for 12–15 minutes, or until golden. Stir in the wine, bay leaves, thyme, sea salt, orange zest and beef stock. Reduce the heat, add the beef cheeks, then cover and cook for 3 hours, or until the cheeks are tender and starting to break apart.

The sauce from the beef cheeks should by now be reduced. If it needs further reducing, remove the cheeks from the pan, cover with foil to keep them warm and simmer the sauce over high heat until nicely reduced. Strain the sauce through a fine sieve and return to the pan. Gently reheat the cheeks in the sauce if necessary whilst preparing the parsnip puree.

Divide the cheeks into deep-bowled plates, cover with the sauce and serve with the parsnip puree and steamed vegetables.

Tips: ~Pre-order beef cheeks from your local butcher. ~To enhance the dish even further, chop some flat leaf parsley, add a little grated orange and finely chop ½ clove of garlic and mix to form a parsley crumb or 'gremolata'. ~Sprinkle the gremolata on the top of the cheeks. ~Don't forget to serve with the meal a glass of the red wine used in the cooking!

Janni's slow cooked shoulder of lamb

Serves 6 • **Prep** 10 mins • **Cook** 6 hrs

2kg shoulder lamb
  (with fat removed
  1.5kg net)
2 tbsp extra virgin oil
2 tsp salt
1 tsp pepper
1 tsp dry Greek oregano
1 tsp ground fennel seeds
12 large green olives, seeded
12 large garlic cloves
1 large lemon, cut into
  8 slices with pips removed
1 large plastic roasting
  oven bag
Risoni pasta
Steamed vegetables or
  Greek salad to serve

Rub lamb with all the ground spices and salt. Place the lamb in a large roasting bag with the lemon and garlic on top, add the olive oil to the top and tie the bag (see photos on following pages). Refrigerate for 1 to 2 hours or overnight to marinate.

Preheat the oven to 130°C. Remove the pips from the olives. Place lamb on a roasting tray and put in the oven (on the middle shelf) and bake for 6 hours, turning once after 4 hours of cooking. To check if the lamb is cooked, remove bag from oven and allow it to cool slightly and wait until the bag deflates. Carefully squeeze the lamb, if it breaks away it is perfectly cooked.

Keep in a warm place. When ready to eat, drain the juices and strain off any excess fat. Serve the juice with the lamb (see photos). Serve with a small pasta such as risoni (orzo), Greek salad or steamed vegetables.

Tips: ~Rather than slow roasting for 6 hours, you can cook the lamb in 2½–3 hours, by cooking it at 160°C. ~The lamb is ideal to reheat for the next day or if there are any leftovers. ~This dish is a great source of protein and iron. ~Ideal for a dinner celebration; also good for a hearty winter lunch.

Story behind the dish: Janni Kyrtsis, my old boss and mentor, came to one of HammondCare's dementia cottages to assist with a Greek-themed dinner celebration. This was his recipe for the dinner and it is truly a memorable lamb dish. PMJ

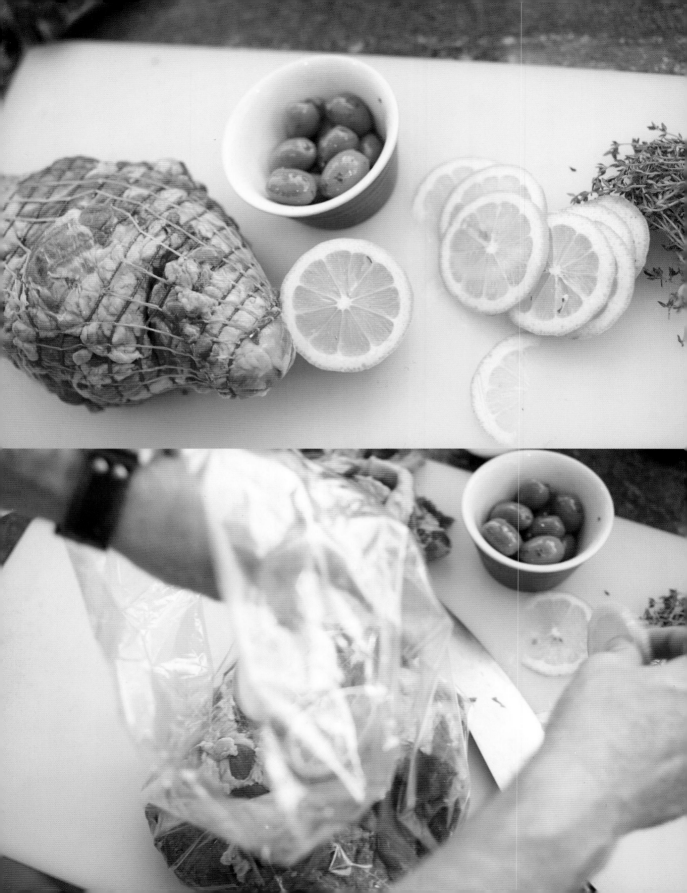

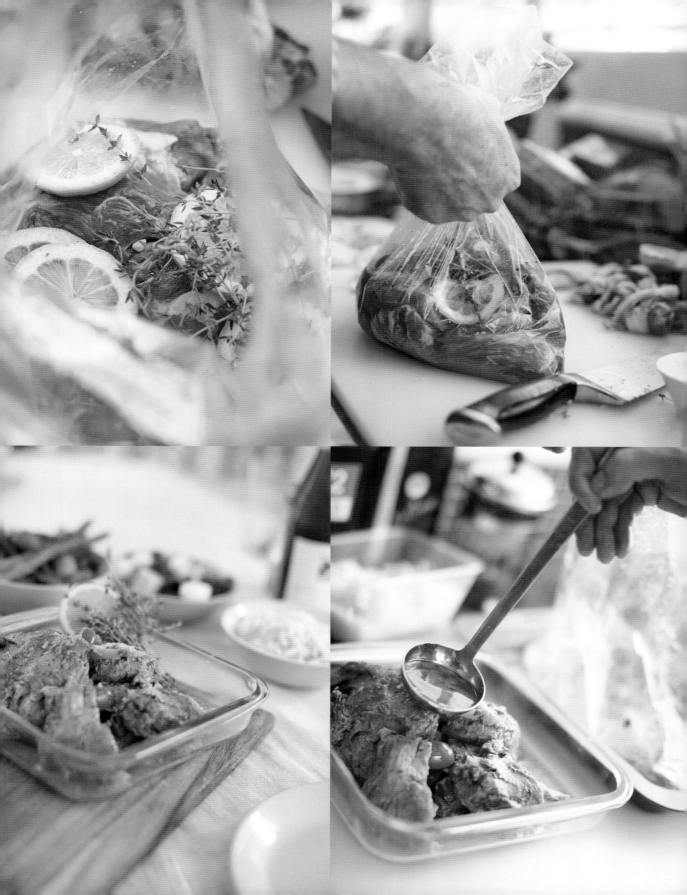

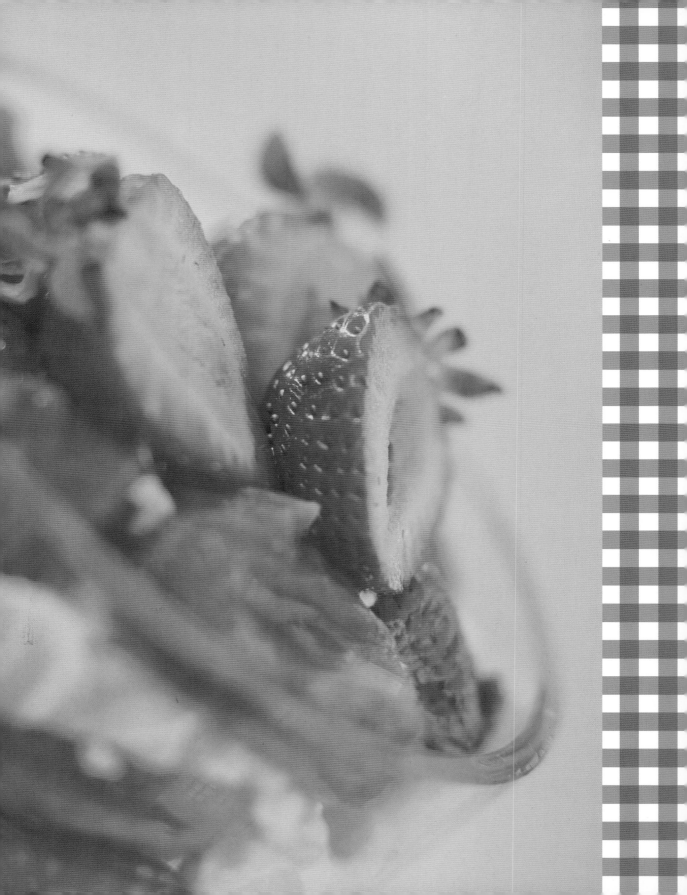

Desserts

What a scrumptious selection of desserts awaits you! Desserts are best when they have a dairy base or are served with half a cup of custard, yoghurt or ice cream. Many of these recipes have been used in HammondCare's residential aged and dementia care, and have been enthusiastically enjoyed!

Cherry jelly cheesecake

Serves 6-8 • **Prep** 30 mins (plus 2½ hours setting time)

Cheesecake mix
400g cream cheese
60g icing sugar
1 tsp vanilla essence
½ tsp ground cinnamon
½ tsp lemon juice
300ml thickened cream

Cherry jelly base
1x 450g Madeira cake
2 tbsp sherry (optional)
½ x 85g raspberry
   jelly packet

Cherry topping
1 small can pitted black
cherries drained
   (reserve liquid)
3 small scoops Gelea Instant
   (see Contacts and resources)

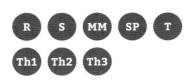

Tips: ~The cheesecake
will keep 24 hours in the
refrigerator, covered. ~The
jelly biscuit can be placed
in glasses or small dessert
bowls, with the cheesecake
filling placed on top.

Line a 20cm springform cake tin with greaseproof paper
or cling wrap. Remove the brown crust from of the Madeira
cake (about 200g). The remainder can be enjoyed with a cup
of tea for a snack. Crumble about 200g of the cake until it
resembles large breadcrumbs and sprinkle onto the lined
springform base. Soak the cake base with 2 tsp sherry
(optional).

Open a small can of pitted black cherries, drain the cherries
and retain the liquid. Place half of an 85g packet of jelly
powder in a bowl and cover with ¾ cup of boiling water and
stir, add ½ cup cold water and stir into the jelly. When the
jelly is made pour into the springform tin covering the cake
crumbs and allow to set in refrigerator until the jelly is firm
(about 1 hour).

Place the cream cheese, icing sugar, vanilla essence and
lemon juice in a bowl and mix thoroughly until smooth and
well combined. In another bowl, whip the cream until firm
and fold through the cream cheese mix. Spoon the cream
cheese topping onto the top of the set jelly base. Cover and
refrigerate for 1 hour.

To make the top of the cheesecake, place 200ml of drained
cherries in the food processor and blend until a smooth
consistency. If a little dry, add a tbsp of the reserved cherry
liquid. Place the blended cherries into a clean small stainless
steel saucepan and add the Gelea Instant. Stir well and bring
to boil, then simmer for 1 minute and remove from heat.

Remove the cheesecake and spread the thickened cherry
puree over the top. Put in refrigerator to set. Remove from
springform tin. Carefully lift away from base and discard the
greaseproof paper or cling wrap. Cut into wedges and serve.

Impossible pie with macerated strawberries

Serves 6-8 • **Prep** 10 mins • **Cook** 1 hr

4 eggs
120g butter
1 cup caster sugar
½ cup self-raising flour
½ tsp salt
½ tsp baking powder
2 cups milk
1 cup desiccated coconut
1 tsp vanilla extract
Custard to serve (about
    400ml)
Macerated strawberries (see
    'Basic recipes')

Preheat oven to 180°C. Grease a 25cm pie dish. Blend all ingredients together until thoroughly mixed. Pour mixture into the pie dish and bake for 1 hour. Remove and serve with custard and macerated strawberries.

Tip: Not too sure how this works, guess it may be magic!

'...carers report people living with dementia grow to prefer sweet foods. Fortunately there are lots of sweet foods high in energy and protein'

Vanilla pannacotta

Serves 4 x 200ml • **Prep** 15 mins (needs to be refrigerated overnight to set) • **Cook** 5 mins

375ml (1½ cups) milk
375ml (1½ cups) cream
80g (⅓ cup) caster sugar
1 tsp vanilla extract
3 x 5g gelatine sheets
Fruit, to serve (see moulded puree fruit recipes for smooth pureed diets)

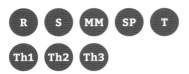

Bring milk, cream, sugar and vanilla to the boil. Remove from heat. Add gelatine and stir until dissolved. Strain liquid, and then pour into 4 x 175 ml ramekins/dariole moulds. Refrigerate overnight.

To serve, use a small spatula or knife to work the pudding away from the edges, then stand moulds in boiling water for 4–5 seconds. Place a plate on top of each mould, then turn over carefully so the plate is on the bottom. Shake to dislodge the pudding. Remove the ramekin and serve with fruit of your choice.

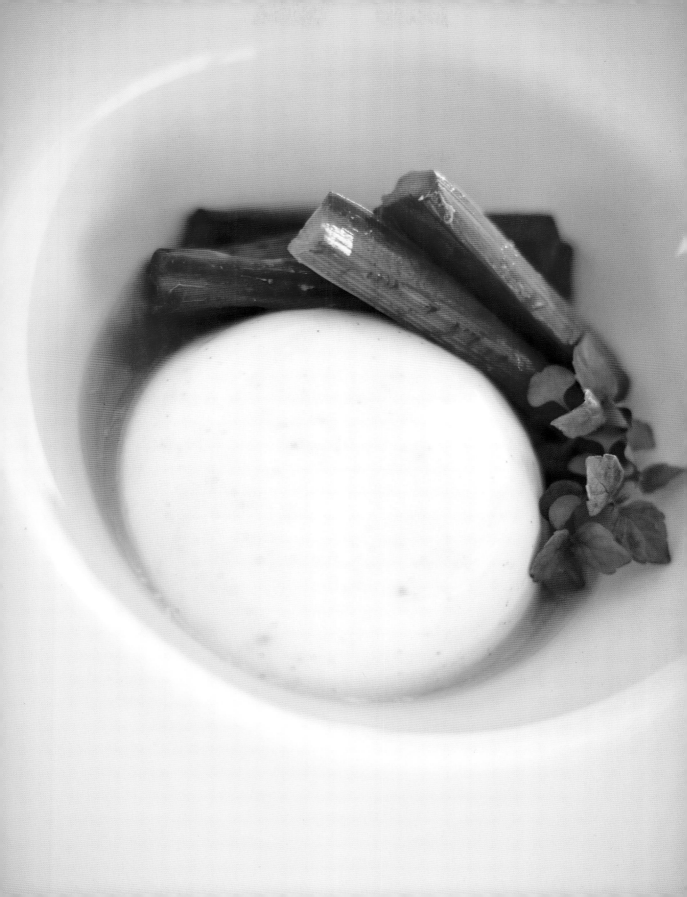

Lemon ricotta cake

Serves 8 • **Prep** 15 mins • **Cook** 45 mins

75g butter
170g caster sugar
100g (1/3 cup) ricotta
3 eggs, separated
175g plain flour
3 tsp baking powder
Grated zest from 1 lemon
50ml fresh lemon juice
30g flaked almonds (garnish)
Icing sugar, to serve
250g ricotta mixed with
    300g vanilla yoghurt to
    serve with cake
1 cup figs or strawberries
    to serve

Preheat oven to 180°C. Grease a 23cm springform tin, then line the bottom with baking paper. Dust tin with a little bit of flour. Cream the butter and sugar together until smooth. Beat in the ricotta.

Beat the egg yolks, add 1 tbsp of the sifted flour, lemon juice and zest and then add to the ricotta mix. Sift remaining flour and baking powder and beat into the ricotta mix until blended sufficiently. Whisk the egg whites until they form peaks. Fold carefully into the ricotta mix using a metal spoon.

Pour into the lined tin and sprinkle the top with the flaked almonds. Bake for 45 minutes at 180°C, remove and allow to cool. Sprinkle with icing sugar and serve with figs or strawberries and blended ricotta and yoghurt.

R T

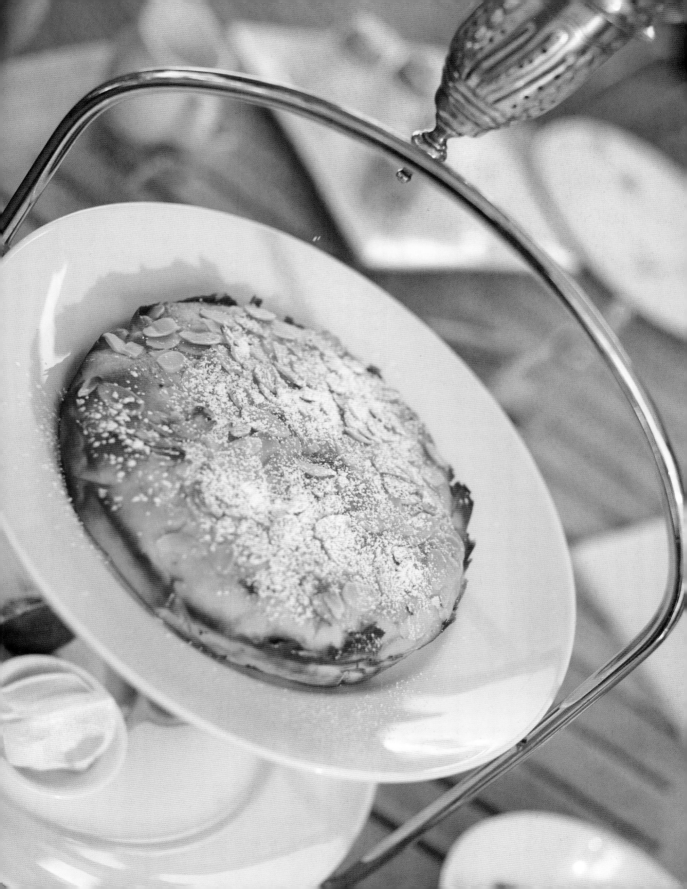

Rich chocolate mousse

Serves 4 • **Prep** 10 mins • **Cook** 8 mins

150g marshmallows,
  chopped in small pieces
60g butter, softened
250g dark chocolate
  (minimum 70 per cent
  cocoa solids), cut into
  small pieces
60ml boiling hot milk
2 tsp dutch cocoa
280ml double cream
1 tsp vanilla extract

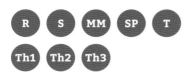

Put the marshmallows, butter, chocolate and milk and cocoa in a heavy-based saucepan. Put the saucepan on the stove, over a low heat, melt the contents, stirring every now and again. Remove from the heat.

Whip the cream with the vanilla extract until thick, and then fold into the cooling chocolate mixture until you have a smooth mixture. Pour into 4 glasses or ramekins (about 175ml or ¾ cup each) and chill until ready to serve.

Tips: ~This is ideal for a smooth pureed diet. ~Also fantastic served with custard and you can also serve with puree fruit, rhubarb, or berry compote. ~For a smooth pureed diet ensure all pureed fruit is thick enough (you may need to use a commercial thickener) and has been passed through a fine sieve to capture any seeds.

Irish rice pudding with sultanas

Serves 4 • **Prep** 10 mins • **Cook** 50 mins

500ml milk
125g thickened cream
1 tsp vanilla essence
1 cinnamon stick
2 cardamom pods, cracked
2 pinches nutmeg
Lemon peel from ½ lemon (no pith)
50g sugar
100g Calrose rice (Australian medium-grain rice)
25g butter
125g mascarpone cheese
4 tbsp sultanas
2 tbsp whiskey

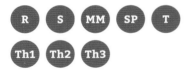

Place the milk, cream, vanilla, cinnamon, lemon zest, cardamom, nutmeg and sugar into a saucepan and bring to boil, then allow to steep for 10 minutes. Remove the cinnamon stick, cardamom and the lemon peel. Add the rice and simmer for 40 minutes.

While the rice is simmering, heat the whiskey with two tablespoons of water in a pan. As soon as it boils remove from the heat and add the sultanas. Allow the sultanas in the syrup (macerated sultanas) to cool. When cool, drain the sultanas.

When the rice is cooked, remove from heat and add the drained, macerated sultanas. Add the butter and fold in the mascarpone.

Tips: ~To make this dish appropriate for someone on moderately thick or extremely thick fluids, just add commercial thickener, following the manufacturer directions for the required consistency, once the butter and mascarpone have been folded through. ~The whiskey can be omitted if you wish to make with no alcohol. ~Heat 50ml of water with 2 tbsp sugar in a saucepan and simmer for 5 minutes. ~Add the sultanas and a drop of vanilla essence and allow to steep. ~If you prefer, you can use sherry or brandy instead of whiskey.

Strawberry Eton mess

Serves 4 • **Prep** 10 mins • **Cook** 10 mins

200ml custard (Use pouring custard and thicken to recommended level)
6 mini-meringues (available at supermarkets)
200ml cream
1 tbsp caster sugar
1 tsp vanilla essence
350g strawberries, hulled and cut into half
1 tbsp icing sugar

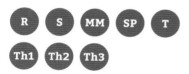

Regular, soft and minced and moist diets
In a bowl, add the cream, caster sugar and vanilla essence. Beat the cream until soft peaks form. Into an 18cm glass bowl (or individual glasses), pour in the thick custard. Crumble the meringues and place half of them on top of the custard.

Cut the strawberries in half, place in a bowl and gently squeeze the juice from them using the back of a spoon. Drain the juice into a cup (retain it for later), then dust the strawberries with the icing sugar, tossing them slightly.

Spoon some of the cream on top of the meringues. Place the squeezed strawberries on top of the cream, place remaining meringue on top of the strawberries and finish off with the remaining cream. Sprinkle with remaining strawberries. Pour the macerated strawberry juice over the top. Serve immediately.

Smooth pureed diet
Crumble the meringue until fine (the best way is to place in a clean plastic bag and bash with a rolling pin until a powder). Prepare the strawberries by placing them in a small stainless steel bowl, add the icing sugar and cover bowl with cling wrap. Place bowl on top of a boiling saucepan of water and simmer for 30–40 minutes, until the strawberries have 'melted'. Allow to cool, then strain through a fine sieve.

Measure the strawberry juice and add commercial thickener, following the manufacturer instructions for required consistency. Blend with stick blender until required consistency achieved.

Place the custard in the bottom of the glass or glasses. Place the whipped cream in a bowl, fold the crushed meringue through the cream, spoon the meringue cream into individual serving dishes and spoon the cooled strawberry puree over the top. Allow to set in fridge for 20 minutes before serving.

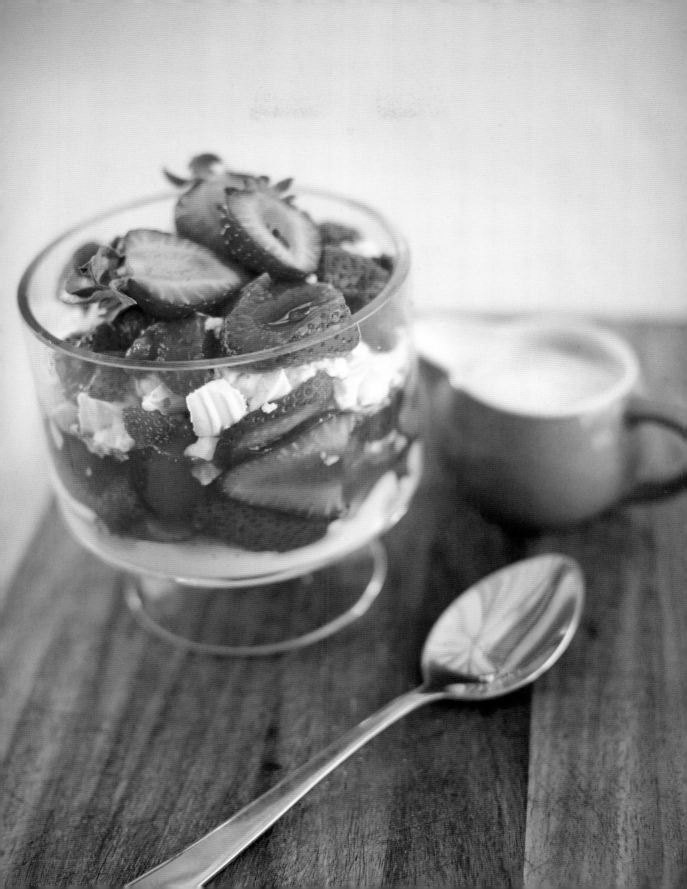

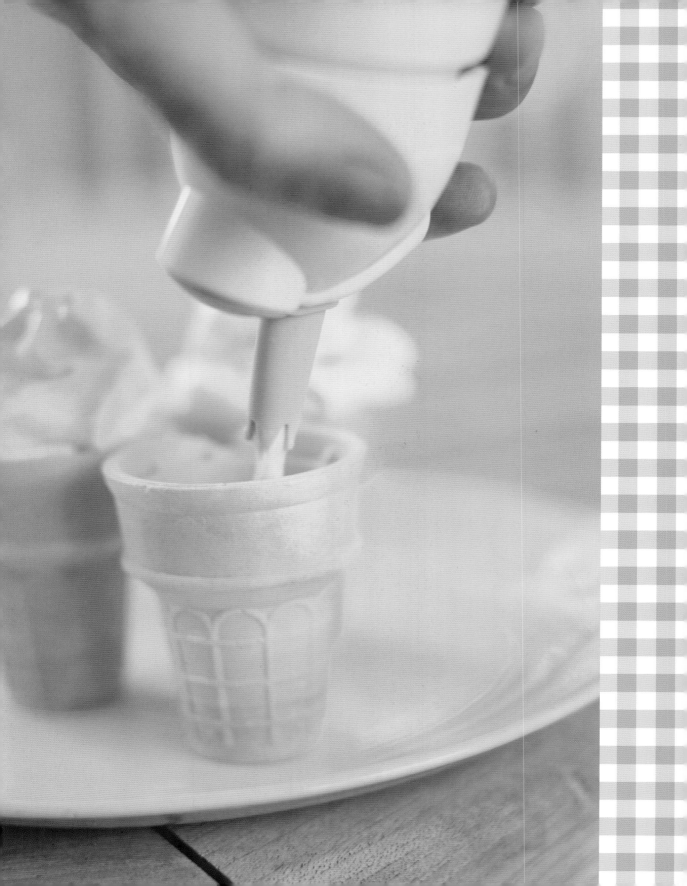

Beverages

Drinks take on a whole new life with our innovative recipes that bring taste and colour to the world of texture-modified diets. Nothing is impossible with a little creativity and care!

Blood orange foam

Serves 1 • **Prep** 2 mins

200ml blood orange juice
(2–3 oranges).
Or normal, freshly squeezed
orange juice.
8 small scoops Spuma
Instant (see 'Contacts and
resources')

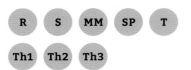

Squeeze oranges and strain through a sieve to ensure all the pulp is left behind. Measure 200ml of juice and add 8 small scoops of Spuma and stir well. Pour into a cream whipping gun and charge with cream whipping bulb (see equipment list). Shake cream whipper for 30 seconds. Pour carefully into glass.

Tips: ~Drinks made with Spuma Instant in a cream whipper look like they contain more fluid than they do because of all the air included to produce the foam. ~The foam in this recipe contains only 200ml of fluid. It is recommended people consume 6–8 cups of fluid per day.

Watermelon, lime and mint foam

Serves 1–2 • **Prep** 5 mins

300g seedless watermelon,
chopped into cubes
Juice of ¼ lemon
6 mint sprigs
8 scoops of Spuma Instant

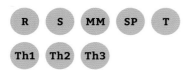

Blend watermelon cubes in a food processor with the lemon juice and mint sprigs. Strain through sieve. Measure 200ml of juice and add 8 small scoops of Spuma. Pour into cream whipping gun and charge with cream whipping bulb (see equipment list). Shake for 30 seconds. Pour carefully into glass.

Green vegetable cocktail

Serves 4 • **Prep** 10 mins

1 cup apple juice
1 ripe avocado (stone and
   skin removed)
1 tbsp continental parsley,
   roughly chopped
1 cup washed baby spinach
   leaves
1 stalk celery, roughly
   chopped
½ Lebanese cucumber,
   seeded and peeled
½ green Granny Smith apple,
   cored and quartered
1 tbsp frozen edamame
   beans (shelled)
½ cm fresh ginger, peeled
Commercial thickener—
   follow manufacturer
   instructions for the
   required consistency

Place all ingredients in a juicer and process, alternatively place in a food blender and strain using a fine conical sieve. For smooth pureed, ensure mixture is lump free. Add the commercial thickeners to a jug, then add the vegetable juice on top and blend with stick blender. Serve in a glass.

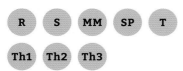

Lemonade

Serves 6 • **Prep** 5 mins

1 cup freshly squeezed
    lemon juice
½ cup caster sugar
4 cups soda water
1 lemon, sliced
1 sprig of mint
Ice cubes

Squeeze the lemon juice , strain through a sieve. Stir in caster sugar and ensure all sugar has dissolved. Pour into glass jug, add sliced lemon and add mint leaves picked from the stem (about 12 leaves). Add the ice cubes and then pour in the chilled soda water. Stir and serve immediately.

For thickened fluid
Ice cubes can be made by thickening water using a commercial thickener to required thickness, pour into ice cube tray and freeze. Make the lemonade without the ice cube, remove the mint and sliced lemon, thicken using a commercial thickener to required thickness. Add thickened ice cubes to lemonade. Pour into glass. Ice cubes are to chill the lemonade and should not be served.

For making a foam
Make the lemonade following main recipe. Pour 200ml of lemonade through a sieve into a bowl. Add 8 small scoops of Spuma Instant, stir well and pour into cream whipper. Charge with cartridge and shake for 30 seconds. Serve in glass for a tasty alternative for a thickened fluid diet. Suitable for all levels of thickness in liquid and food.

Grilled grapefruit and cherry foam

Serves 1-2 • **Prep** 2 mins • **Cook** 5 mins

2 grapefruit (for 200ml
  grapefruit juice)
2 tsp palm sugar or soft
  brown sugar
1 tsp cinnamon
1 pinch ground ginger
  (optional)
½ tsp vanilla extract
  (optional)
10 hulled cherries
8 small scoops Spuma
  Instant
Orange or apple juice (in
  case not enough juice
  from the grapefruits)

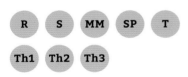

Wash grapefruit and cut it in half, along the hemisphere. Use a small knife to cut around the outside of the grapefruit (between the fruit and the pith—the white part—then cut along each of the white membranes separating the sections. This will make it much easier to scoop out the fruit later. On top of each grapefruit half, evenly sprinkle the sugar, cinnamon, ginger and vanilla.

Heat a non-stick pan on medium high heat. Place the grapefruit face down on the pan. Grill for 2-3 minutes, making sure not to burn. Alternatively, place the grapefruit under a grill until the sugar is bubbling. Allow the grapefruit to cool.

Remove the pips and place 10 cherries in a food processor/ blender. Squeeze the grapefruits through a fine sieve, retaining 2 of the grapefruit skin shells. Measure 200ml of the grapefruit liquid. If a little short it can be topped up with apple juice or orange juice.

Pour the 200ml of strained grapefruit juice into the blender with the cherries and blend well. Strain the grapefruit liquid and mix in 8 scoops of Spuma Instant. Stir and pour into cream whipping gun. Charge with cream whipping bulb. Shake for 30 seconds. Pour foam into the two halves of grapefruit skin and serve immediately.

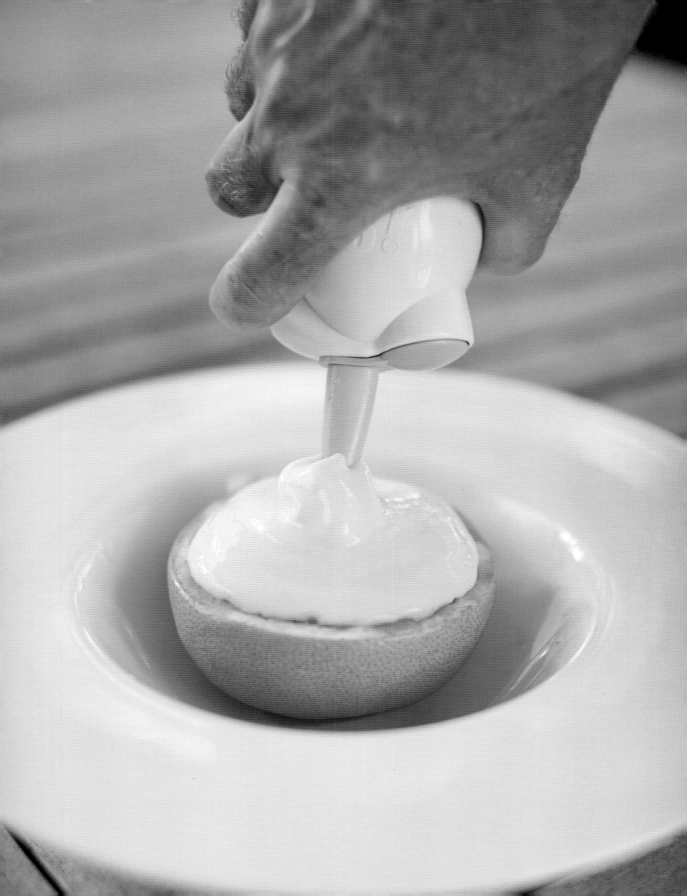

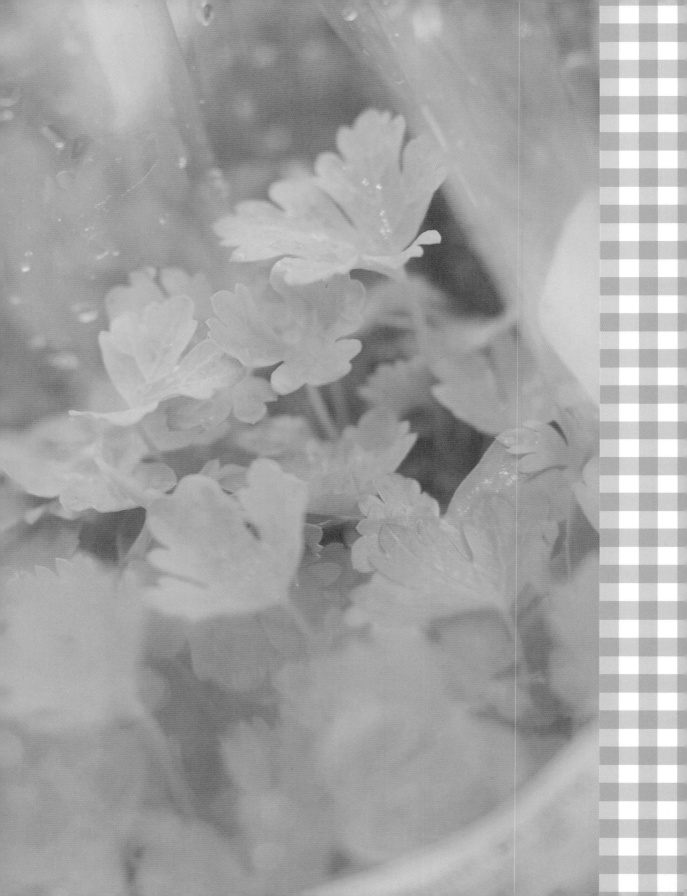

Soft

Some people have been given a clinical recommendation for a soft diet. For our team, that's not a reason to miss out on great meals! The following recipes are ideal for lunch or dinner and will tempt taste buds while being safe for people on soft diets. They complement the many options in other recipe sections where the soft symbol is seen.

Spanish omelette with wilted spinach

Serves 2–3 • **Prep** 12 mins • **Cook** 8 mins

1 onion, finely sliced
4 small boiled chat potatoes, skin removed and diced
2 large tomatoes—skinned, seeded and chopped
2 tsp olive oil
120g shredded cheese (mozzarella or Gruyere)
4 eggs
2 tsp cream
1 tsp chopped parsley
½ tsp of chopped thyme
250g washed baby spinach
Sea salt and pepper to taste

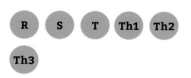

Using a small omelette pan, gently fry onion and potato in 1 tbsp of olive oil until golden brown, frequently turning the mixture. Add tomato and fry for a further 3 minutes. Lightly beat eggs with cream and parsley, then season with salt and pepper. Pour over vegetables in omelette pan and sprinkle with the cheese.

Cook gently until omelette has firmed on bottom. Brown under grill for about 30 seconds, until the top has just set. Cut into half and serve two plates by sliding unfolded onto the plate.

Heat 1 tbsp olive oil in a frying pan, when hot add the English spinach and allow to wilt, stirring throughout. Season with salt and pepper, remove from pan with tongs, squeezing out any moisture and place next to the omelette.

Skinning tomatoes
Remove the core stem from the tomato. Place in a small pan of boiling water for 30 seconds or until skin starts peeling off. Remove and place in iced water, take off skin and cut tomato in half, removing seeds.

Tips: ~Any soft combinations can be added to the omelette. ~Bacon dust can be sprinkled onto the omelette for more flavour (see 'Basic recipes'). ~High in calcium because of the cheese and a good source of protein.

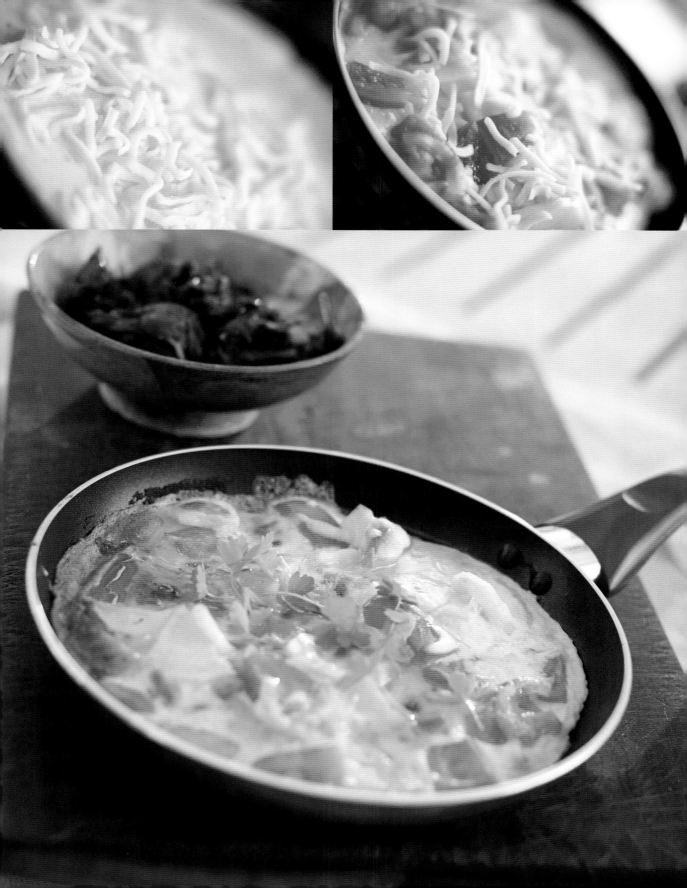

Risoni with bolognaise sauce

Serves 4 • **Prep** 15 mins • **Cook** 45 mins

400g minced veal (or beef)
1 carrot, peeled
1 celery rib, stringy fibres
    removed
100ml olive oil
½ brown onion
1 garlic clove crushed and
    chopped finely
½ cup tomato paste
2 tbsp flour
½ cup red wine
500ml beef stock (see Basic
    recipes or purchase ready-
    made stock)
¾ tsp ground white pepper
1 tsp salt
Bouquet garni (a sprig of
    rosemary, thyme, 4 parsley
    stalks and 2 bay leaves
    tied together with string or
    muslin cloth)
100g Parmesan cheese,
    grated
250g packet risoni

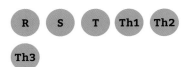

Chop the celery, carrot and onion in a food processer until finely chopped, heat ½ the oil and cook the vegetables for 5 minutes, remove the vegetables and heat remaining oil in frying pan. Add the veal or beef mince to the pan and fry until golden, stirring to separate the mince, then add the flour to bind the mince. Add the garlic, cooked vegetables, tomato paste and red wine to the pan and stir well. Simmer for 2 minutes.

Remove mince and vegetables from frying pan and place into a stainless steel saucepan, add the stock and seasoning, and bring to the boil, removing any scum from the surface with a slotted spoon. Turn down the heat and add the bouquet garni. Allow the bolognaise to simmer for 40 minutes, skimming occasionally to remove any impurities.

Place a small stainless steel pot on the stove and fill with 1.5 litres of water, add a dash of olive oil and season with salt. When the water is boiling, add the risoni and cook for 6–8 minutes or until tender. Drain the risoni pasta, add 1 tbsp olive oil and season with salt and pepper. Divide the pasta into 4 bowls and spoon the bolognaise sauce on top. Add the Parmesan cheese on top. Ensure that it has melted before serving.

For those on thickened fluids: serve the sauce with a slotted spoon to drain off any liquid. If you wish to serve with additional sauce ensure this is thickened with a commercial thickener.

Tips: 150g cooked peas can also be incorporated into the bolognaise for added flavour.

Italian sausage and cannellini bean casserole with tomatoes

Serves 2–3 • **Prep** 10 mins • **Cook** 20 mins

4 Italian sausages
1 x 400g can cannellini beans
1 x 400g can diced tomatoes
300ml beef stock (see Basic
  recipes) or purchase
  ready-made variety
½ tsp fennel seeds
1 garlic clove, crushed
½ onion, chopped
1 pinch chilli powder
1 carrot, peeled and diced
100g frozen peas
1 tbsp olive oil
1 tbsp chopped parsley
Sea salt and pepper to taste

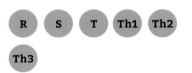

Remove the skins from the sausages and crumble the sausage meat. Heat oil in a large stainless steel saucepan and cook the onion until translucent, add the garlic, then the sausage crumbs and finally the diced carrot, allow the sausage meat to turn brown.

Wash and drain well the cannellini beans. Add the tomatoes, fennel seeds, cannellini beans, beef stock and chilli to the saucepan and simmer for 15 minutes. Finally add the peas and simmer for another 5 minutes, adjust the seasoning and add the chopped parsley.

Tips: ~This is a great hearty meal, budget friendly and will freeze well. ~If preparing for people on thickened fluids, serve with a slotted spoon and ensure any sauce is thickened with a commercial thickener to the required consistency.

Steamed barramundi with ratatouille

Serves 2 • **Prep** 10 mins • **Cook** 20 mins

2 x 120g portions of barramundi (skin on)
1 lemon
⅓ cup Spanish onion, diced (about 50g)
100g tinned diced tomatoes
1 zucchini, diced in 1cm cubes (about 100g)
½ small eggplant diced in 1 cm cubes (about 100g)
1 red capsicums, diced in 1cm cubes (about 100g)
½ cup olive oil
1 garlic clove, crushed
1½ tsp salt
½ tsp pepper
Sprig of thyme
1 tbsp chopped parsley
Creamed potato to serve (see Basic recipes)

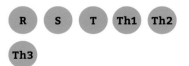

Place steamer basket on a wok or large saucepan half filled with water. Ensure the basket covers the saucepan or wok. Bring to simmer until steam is coming out of the basket. In a stainless steel saucepan slowly cook the diced Spanish onion in the olive oil until translucent. Add the garlic and eggplant and tomatoes. Season and simmer covered for 10 minutes, remove lid and add a sprig of thyme and the zucchini. Cover and simmer until vegetables are cooked. Add the chopped parsley and taste for seasoning. Keep warm and cook fish.

Place the two portions of Barramundi skin-side down on buttered baking paper into the steamer, cover with steamer basket lid until fish is cooked (about 10 minutes). Check after 5 minutes to ensure the water has not evaporated, top upwith boiling water. Carefully remove the fish with a fish slice and place on top of the warm ratatouille on two plates.

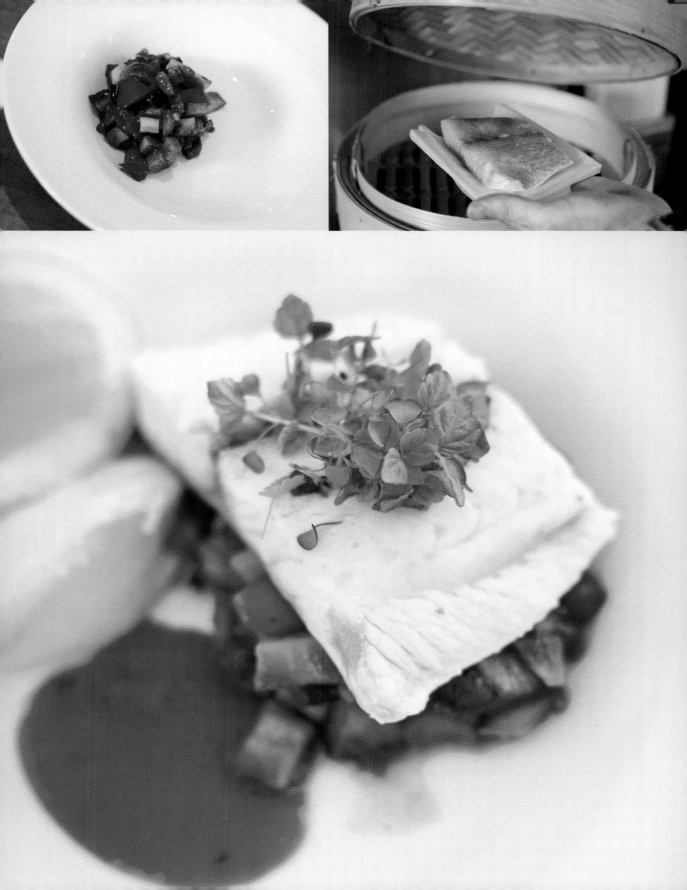

Cottage pie

Serves 3 • **Prep** 15 mins • **Cook** 50 mins

1 tbsp olive oil
300g lean lamb mince
½ onion, finely diced
½ carrot, finely diced
½ celery stick, chopped
1 garlic clove, finely chopped
1 tbsp plain flour
2 tsp tomato paste
50ml red wine
300ml beef stock
1 tbsp Worcestershire sauce
1 sprig of thyme
1 bay leaf
½ tsp sea salt
1 pinch pepper

Mash
500g potatoes, peeled and
    chopped
60ml cream
3 tsp butter
2 tbsp cheddar cheese,
    grated
1 pinch of nutmeg
Salt and ground white
    pepper to taste
Chopped chives for garnish
    (optional)

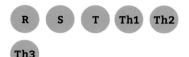

Heat oil in a large saucepan and fry the mince until browned. Remove the cooked meat. Put the rest of the oil into the pan, add the vegetables and cook on a gentle heat until soft (about 20 minutes). Add the garlic, flour and tomato paste, increase the heat and cook for 3 minutes, then return the beef to the pan.

Pour over the wine, and boil to reduce it slightly before adding the stock, Worcestershire sauce, thyme and bay leaf. Bring to a simmer and cook, uncovered, for 20 minutes. Check after about 10 minutes—if a lot of liquid remains, increase the heat slightly to reduce the sauce. After 20 minutes the sauce should be thick and coating the meat.

Season well and then discard the bay leaf and thyme sprig. Serve with a slotted spoon and ensure no thin fluids are given to those recommended thickened fluids. Thicken with a commercial thickener if required.

Mash
Peel the potatoes and cut up into equal size pieces. Cook in salted water until soft. Drain the salted water and add cream and butter. Pass through a mouli or ricer or mash until no lumps. Season to taste and sprinkle in the grated cheese.

Assemble the cottage pie
Preheat oven to 180°C. Place the lamb mince into a small ovenproof casserole dish or divide into 3 small ovenproof individual casserole dishes about 130–140g per serve. Cover with the mash.

Cover the cottage pie with foil (stops the top crusting) and place in oven and heat for 15 minutes at 180°C. Place a clean digital thermometer inside the pie. It should read 75°C when heated through. Serve with steamed green vegetables (cooked to be soft).

Story behind the dish: This recipe was inspired and adapted from a recipe I cooked for a young prince in Highgrove House. PMJ

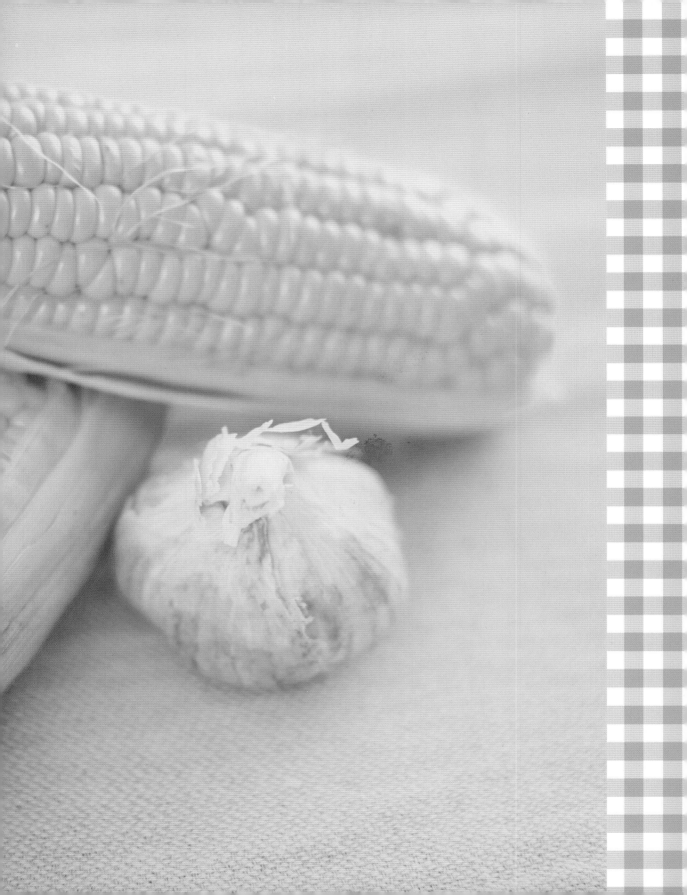

Minced & moist

Minced and moist may not sound the most appetising diet but for many people, it is essential for their well-being.

Even if food needs to be finely diced and moist for easy swallowing, it can still be spectacular, as our special selection of recipes shows. And there are many other recipes featuring the featuring the minced and moist symbol throughout *Don't give me eggs that bounce.*

Pizza soufflé

Serves 2 • **Prep** 10 mins • **Cook** 40 mins

100g grated mozzarella
6 slices of bread, crust
  removed
¾ cup milk
80g ham, finely chopped
  in a food processor
½ cup tomato sauce
  (see Basic recipes) or
  tomato passata
¼ tsp chopped oregano
¼ tsp chopped basil
2 eggs
1 tbsp grated Parmesan
  cheese
2 tsp butter
Sea salt and pepper

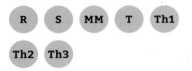

Soak the bread slices in milk for 10 minutes. Drain the excess. Preheat oven to 180°C. Line the bottom of a small casserole dish with ½ of the bread slices, top with ⅓ of the tomato sauce/passata, sprinkle with some of the herbs and ½ of the ham. Add a layer of ½ of the mozzarella. Season with salt and pepper.

Repeat process and cover with tomato sauce/passata, oregano, ham and mozzarella. Add a layer of the remaining bread slices. Beat the eggs with the Parmesan. Prick the bread layer with a fork all over and pour the egg mixture on top. Coax the egg to absorb into the holes of the bread slices until totally absorbed.

Cut the butter into pieces and sprinkle over the top of the soufflé. Put soufflé in the preheated oven. Cook for 40 minutes covered. Crusty parts are not suitable for a soft or minced and moist diet. Any formed crust needs to be removed before serving.

For those on thickened fluids, ensure any fluid is thickened with a commercial thickener to the appropriate consistency.

Tips: This is a great source of protein and calcium.

Story behind the dish: This started as a cooking challenge at home with my daughter Cristabel. We worked together to make this dish. PMJ

Seafood chowder

Serves 2 • **Prep** 15 mins • **Cook** 25 mins

½ tbsp olive oil
½ onion, finely chopped in
   food processor
1 tbsp bacon dust (see
   Basic recipes)
½ tbsp plain flour
300ml fish stock (ready-made)
120g Desiree potato, peeled
   and finely diced (0.5cm)
Pinch of nutmeg
Pinch of cayenne pepper
150ml milk
100g boneless white fish,
   chopped in food processor
60g green prawn meat,
   peeled and chopped in
   food processor
4 tbsp thickened cream
50g cooked mussels (or
   equivalent cooked shellfish
   such as tinned smoked
   oysters, clams), chopped
   in food processor
100g carrots, finely diced (0.5cm)
30–40g crustless white fresh
   breadcrumbs
1 tbsp parsley, finely chopped
Sea salt and ground white
   pepper to taste

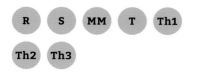

Heat the oil in a large saucepan over a medium heat, and then add the processed onion, carrot and bacon. Cook for 8 mins until the onion is soft and the bacon is cooked. Stir in the flour, then cook for a further 2 mins.

Pour in the fish stock and bring it up to a gentle simmer. Add the small diced potatoes, cover, then simmer for 5 minutes until the potatoes are cooked through. Add the ground nutmeg, cayenne pepper and salt and pepper to taste, then stir in the milk.

Process the mussels and prawn meat in a food processor, storing it in the fridge for later use. Process the white fish in a food processor, then gently simmer the fish in the fish stock for 4 minutes. Add the cream and shellfish (mussels and prawns), then simmer for 1 minute more. Check the seasoning and add salt and pepper to taste.

Remove the crust from white bread and process in food processor, until a fine white bread crumb is achieved. Carefully add small portions of the breadcrumbs, stirring until the liquid thickens to the right consistency. Add a commercial thickener to thicken the chowder to the appropriate consistency if required. Sprinkle with the finely chopped parsley and serve.

Tips: ~Any combination of shellfish can be used. Tinned mussels and oysters are a great shelf stable option for enhancing seafood soups. ~If using canned oysters or clams drain the meat and run under cold water to remove the preserving liquid. ~The fish can also be swapped for smoked fish salmon or ocean trout (ensure no bones). ~A good source of calcium.

Chicken and corn soup with herb butter

Serves 6 as an entree • **Prep** 10 mins • **Cook** 20 mins

*Garlic butter (makes enough
for 8–10 portions)*
2 cloves garlic
80g butter
1½ tbsp Italian parsley,
  chopped
1 tsp chives, finely snipped
¼ tsp ground cumin

Soup
4 corn cobs or 350g of frozen *2 c.*
  corn kernels, defrosted
150g chicken, finely diced *3 lbs*
  (no more than 0.5cm
  pieces)
1.25lt chicken stock *5 cups*
50g butter *3.5 tbsp.*
1 clove garlic, finely chopped
Sea salt and ground white
  pepper to taste

Garlic butter
Soften the butter. Fold in all the ingredients and stir. Wrap into a cylinder (20 cent coin diameter) using cling wrap and chill.

Soup
Remove husks from the corncobs and using a knife, cut all kernels off the cob, by sliding the knife down four sides of the corn. Melt the butter, sweat off the onions and garlic for 4 minutes—no colour. Add 1 litre of stock and bring to boil. Add the freshly husked corn kernels, cover and simmer until cooked (about 15 minutes). Add the chicken and simmer for a further 5 minutes. Remove from the heat and use a stick blender to puree the mixture until smooth. Season with salt and pepper. Use a commercial thickener to ensure the appropriate consistency for those on thickened fluids.

Serve hot with a 0.5cm thin slice of garlic butter on top.

Tips: Ideal served chilled on a hot summer's day and is great as an addition to an afternoon tea.

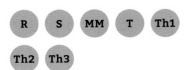

(R) (S) (MM) (T) (Th1)
(Th2) (Th3)

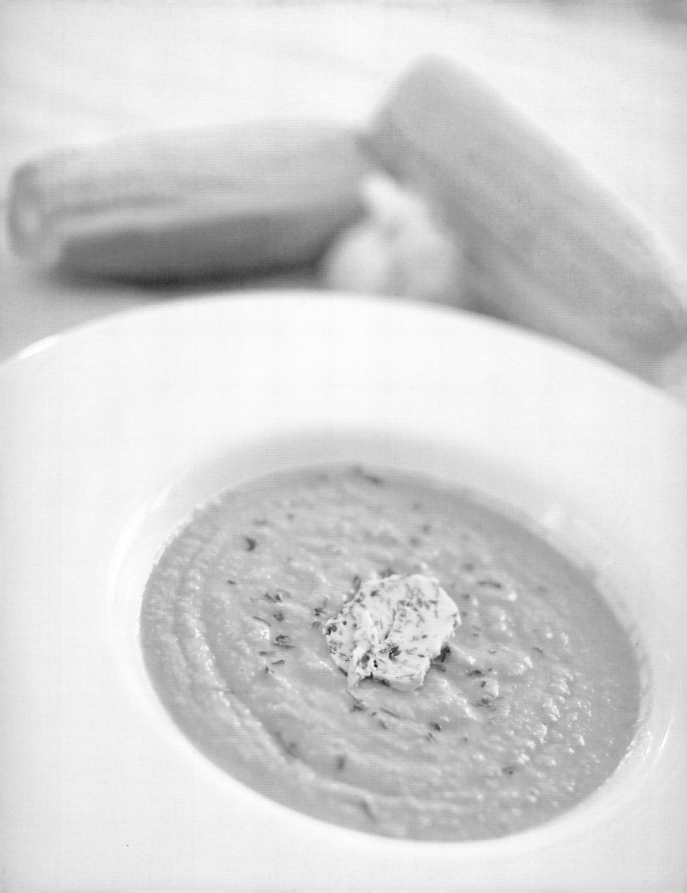

Boston baked beans, scrambled egg and bacon dust

Serves 2 • **Prep** 10 mins • **Cook** 60 mins

Boston baked beans
½ tbsp olive oil
1 clove garlic
1 x 400g can of cannellini beans
100g diced bacon (0.5cm)
½ brown onion, finely diced
    (0.5 cm)
½ x 400g can of diced
    tomato, diced finely (0.5cm)
½ tbsp Worcestershire sauce
1 tbsp soft brown sugar
1 tbsp golden syrup
2 tsp Dijon mustard (mild)
1 cup vegetable or beef stock
2 tsp tomato powder—
    available from Herbie's
Spices online shop (optional)
Sea salt and ground white
    pepper to taste

Scrambled eggs
(see Breakfast recipes)
2 eggs
3 tbsp cream
2 tsp butter
Sea salt
Ground white pepper

Bacon dust
(see 'Basic recipes' for
method)
4 rashers of bacon, very thin

Follow recipe to make bacon dust. To make the baked beans, place olive oil into a heavy bottom saucepan and add the onion, garlic and bacon, cook until slightly coloured but not brown (3–4 minutes). Add beans (drained and washed), tomato, golden syrup, mustard, Worcestershire sauce, sugar and 1 cup of stock and tomato powder. Bring to the boil, then transfer to ovenproof casserole dish. Bake, covered, for 30 minutes at 180°C. Remove cover and stir. Bake for a further 20–30 minutes or until thickened. Follow recipe (breakfast recipes) to make scrambled egg.

To serve the meal, place a generous amount of Boston baked beans into 2 ceramic bowls, divide scrambled egg into another 2 ceramic serving bowls. Finally add 1 tbsp of bacon dust into 2 small ceramic bowls. Place the three dishes on rectangle serving plates.

Tips: ~Can also be served with soaked bread (suitable for a minced and moist diet). ~This dish can be modified for smooth pureed diet (see recipe for scrambled eggs in breakfast to guide you through the process for scrambled egg puree). ~The dust is safe to use as long as it is folded well into the puree before eating. ~The reason for separating the three dishes is to enable flavour separation, rather than creating a one-pot wonder blend.

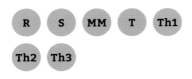

Story behind this dish: It was created for Bob from Woy Woy, who had a narrowed oesophagus and found it hard to eat. He had a craving for bacon, eggs and baked beans. I wanted to encapsulate all the flavours for him in a way that met his craving. PMJ

Lentil soup with crumbled sausage

Serves 2 • **Prep** 10 mins • **Cook** 30 mins

200g Italian sausages (about 2½ thin sausages), skin removed and finely chopped (0.5 cm)
1 tbsp olive oil
½ Spanish onion, finely diced (0.5cm)
1 clove garlic chopped
1 carrot, peeled and finely diced
1 small zucchini, finely diced
1 tsp ground cumin
2 cups beef stock
3 tbsp red wine
1 small tomato, seeds removed and finely diced
100g green lentils (French style)
2 tsp chopped continental parsley
Sea salt and pepper to taste
1 slice sourdough bread, crust removed and crumbled into small pieces

Heat the oil in a stainless steel pot, add the chopped onion and carrot and simmer for 5 minutes. Add the sausage into the oil and brown the meat, then add the garlic and cook for 2 minutes. Add flour and stir for 2 more minutes.

Add the lentils, stock and wine and simmer for 15 minutes or until the lentils are cooked. Do not season until lentils are cooked. Add the zucchini and simmer for 5 minutes. Season the soup to taste, then add the tomato, chopped parsley and cumin. Add a commercial thickener, following the manufacturer instructions for those on thickened fluids.

Divide the bread into two bowls, and pour the soup on top. Allow bread to soak in the soup before serving.

Tips: ~Canned lentils can be used to replace the green lentils, just drain, wash and add ⅓ of can to broth at the same time you add the zucchini.
~A budget-friendly soup, high in protein.

(R) (S) (MM) (T) (Th1)
(Th2) (Th3)

Moroccan lamb, sultanas and green olives

Serves 2–3 • **Prep** 10 mins • **Cook** 70 mins

½ tbsp olive oil
400g diced or minced lamb
   (0.5cm diced)
250ml (1 cup) beef stock
½ brown onion, finely diced
   (0.5cm)
½ tsp chopped garlic
1 tbsp Moroccan spice
400g can of lentils, drained
   and roughly chopped
   (about 260g)
Zest from 2 oranges
   –pith off
2 bay leaves
1 tbsp sultanas chopped fine
1 tbsp chopped coriander
2 tbsp Greek yoghurt (omit
   for those on thickened
   fluids)
2 tbsp green olives, finely
   chopped (0.5cm)
Sea salt and pepper to taste

Couscous
¾ cup couscous
¾ cup beef stock
1 tbsp orange juice
1 tsp butter
¼ tsp cumin

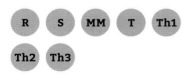

Brown the onions in half of the olive oil in a heavy based saucepan, add the garlic and cook—do not allow to burn. Remove onion and garlic from the saucepan and then add the rest of the oil to the saucepan and heat.

Add the meat to the oil and stir until all the meat has browned. Add the stock and garlic and onion mixture to the meat. Bring to a simmer and then add the bay leaves, chopped olives and lentils, then cover and cook for 60 minutes on a slow heat until the meat is tender.

Meanwhile make the couscous, by bringing ¾ cup stock to the boil. Place the couscous and stock into a small stainless steel bowl or heatproof glass bowl. Add the butter, cumin and orange juice and cover with a tight fitting lid or cling wrap. Allow the couscous to steep for 5 mins, remove lid or wrap and flake with a fork to separate grains.

Remove lid from meat and season with sea salt and ground black pepper, then add the sultanas and simmer for 5 more minutes, before adding the chopped coriander.

Ensure the lamb mix is reduced to correct consistency for a minced and moist diet. Serve with the couscous and a generous dollop of yoghurt.

For those on thickened fluids, ensure you serve with a slotted spoon and thicken any liquid to the appropriate consistency. Omit yoghurt.

Tips: Ensure the couscous is adequately soaked with the Moroccan lamb sauce before serving.

Chilli con carne

Serves 2 • **Prep** 10 mins • **Cook** 45 mins

1 tbsp olive oil
300g lean beef mince
½ Spanish onion, finely
   diced (0.5 cm)
½ red capsicum, finely diced
1 clove garlic, chopped finely
1½ cups beef stock
400g can diced tomato
1 tsp ground cumin
1 tsp ground coriander
1 tbsp tomato paste
1 tsp paprika
¼ tsp chilli powder
   (add to taste)
Sea salt and pepper to taste

Refried beans
   (see Basic recipes)

Guacamole
   (see Basic recipes)

In a saucepan heat the oil and brown the onion, add the beef mince and break down with a spoon until it turns into a crumbled, golden brown consistency. Blend the diced tomatoes in the food processor (or with a stick blender) and add to the onions.

Add the rest of the ingredients except the capsicum and simmer for 20 minutes. Add the capsicum and simmer for a further 20 minutes, stirring frequently ensuring it doesn't stick on the bottom. Serve with a slotted spoon and ensure no unmodified fluids are given to those on thickened fluids. Thicken with a commercial thickener if required.

Tips: ~Serve with refried beans, guacamole and chopped coriander. ~A good source of fibre, iron and protein.

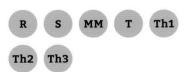

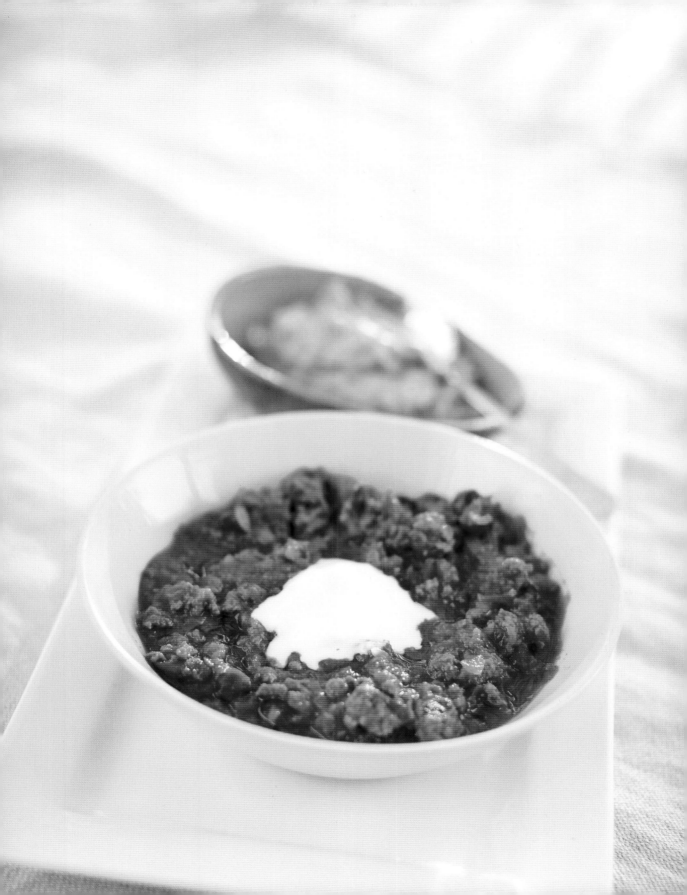

Beef, shiraz and mushroom casserole

Serves 2–4 • **Prep** 10 mins • **Cook** 45 mins

1 tbsp olive oil
400g lean beef mince
½ onion chopped fine
½ tbsp tomato paste
1 small carrot, peeled and chopped fine (0.5cm)
100g field mushrooms, chopped fine
2 tsp porcini mushroom dust (see basic recipes) —optional
2 tbsp plain flour
300ml beef stock (see basic recipes)
150ml (1 cup) shiraz
1 bouquet garni (½ bunch thyme, 2 bay leaves and a few parsley stalks tied together)
100g bacon finely chopped (0.5cm)

Pea puree
 (see Basic recipes)
  —serving suggestions

Creamed potato
(see Basic recipes)
  —serving suggestion

Heat half the oil in a stainless steel pan, brown the mince, then set aside. Add the onions and carrots to the pan, adding a drizzle more oil, then cook on a low heat for 5 mins until coloured.

Add the bacon and stir well, sprinkle in the porcini mushroom powder (optional), then add the flour. Add the mince back in with the vegetables. Add the field mushrooms and tomato paste and pour in the red wine and beef stock. Bring to boil and then turn down to a simmer; skim the surface removing any scum.

Cover pan with a lid and cook for 30 minutes or until the meat is tender. If it is drying out, add a little more stock. Remove bouquet garni. When cooked, remove from heat and serve with creamed potato and pea puree. Ensure this is served with a slotted spoon or that all liquids are thickened to the appropriate consistency.

Tips: ~High in protein and fibre, if served with a pea puree. ~For a regular diet, you can add a crust.

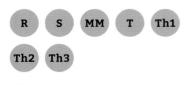

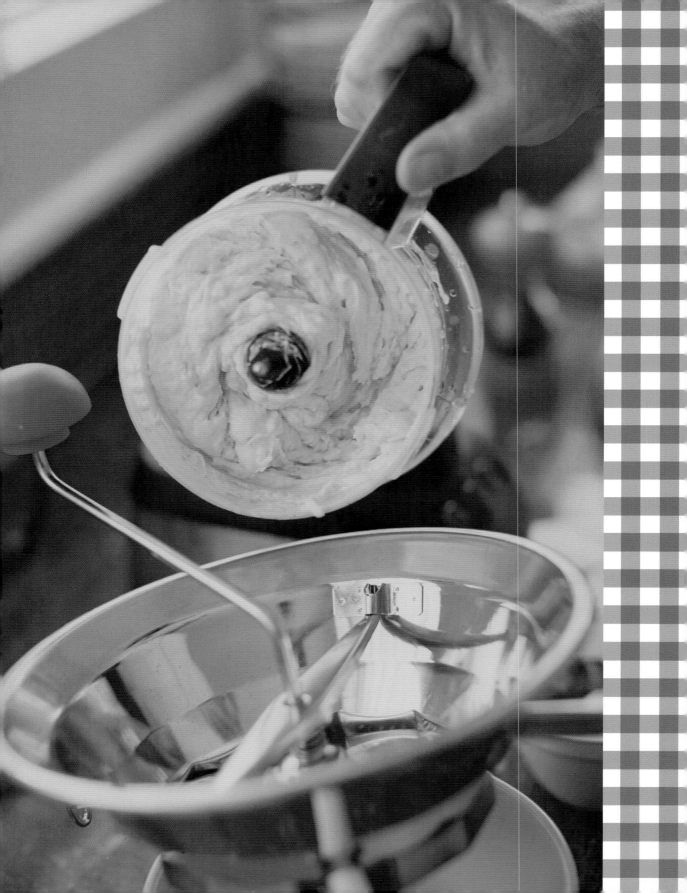

Smooth pureed

Many people with dementia and other conditions are unable to swallow food of any consistency beyond smooth pureed. This can sometimes be disheartening, not just for the person eating but also for those preparing and serving.

A special focus for our chef Peter Morgan-Jones has been to restore dignity and lift morale through creative smooth pureed dishes, with separation of flavours and amazing presentation.

Many a smile has greeted these dishes and we are sure this will be your experience too as you share the joy of smooth pureed food.

Semolina pizza with ricotta and basil

Serves 2 (makes 3 x 31cm pizzas, about 1.5 pizzas = 1 serve)
• **Prep** 10 mins • **Cook** about 5–8 mins

500ml milk
120ml fine semolina
50g finely grated Parmesan
   cheese
1 tsp ground white pepper
1½ tsp sea salt
1 egg yolk
20g butter
Extra good quality Parmesan
   for building pizza and
   serving

Topping
150g ricotta
3 tsp tomato paste
Basil pesto (recipe below)

Pesto
20 basil leaves
1 tsp shaved Parmesan
1 tsp almond meal
2 tbsp extra virgin olive oil
½ clove garlic

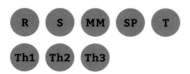

Heat the milk in a stainless steel pan, add the semolina in a fine stream, stirring constantly with a wooden spoon. Stir until smooth (about 3 minutes on high heat). Remove from heat and add the seasoning, butter, Parmesan and egg yolk, stirring until it is all incorporated and glossy.

Line a tray with baking paper and pour mixture onto the paper. With a pastry scraper/spatula smooth out the mixture until it is 1cm thick. Allow to cool and refrigerate until set.

Make the pesto
Place all pesto ingredients in a small food processor and blend until a smooth paste, alternatively place in a cup and use stick blender to turn into a paste, add a little more oil if it is dry. Ensure there are no lumps in the pesto.

Assemble the pizza
Season the ricotta with sea salt and a little ground white pepper. Using a knife or a cutter, cut the semolina slab into 3 round discs (about 30cm diameter)—don't worry if it only makes two, retain all the cutting scraps and form into a 1 cm thick circle and use knife/cutter again.

On each semolina pizza base spread 1 tsp of tomato paste until evenly coated, then place about 50g of ricotta and a generous spoonful of pesto. Finely grate Parmesan over each pizza base (using a micro plane grater)—about 2 tsp per pizza base will give a nice amount of flavour. Drizzle a little olive oil on top.

recipe continues...

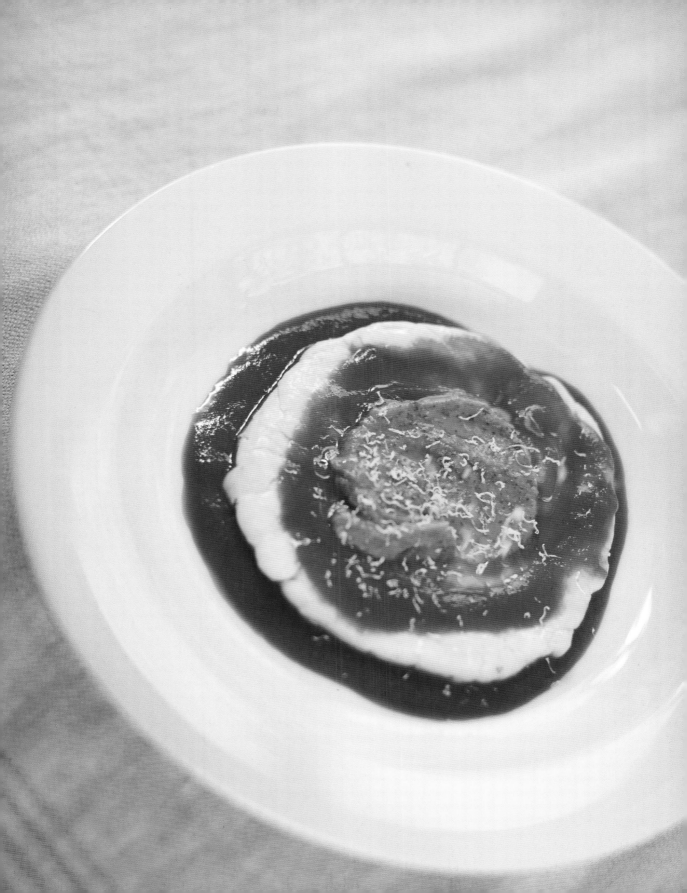

Semolina pizza with ricotta and basil

To serve

Place pizza onto a serving plate, cover with cling wrap and microwave on high for 1 minute or until pizza is heated through. Alternatively it can be heated in oven at 100°C for 15 minutes as long as it is covered in foil. Any crisp edges or crusty pieces need to be removed to be suitable for a soft, minced and moist or smooth pureed diet.

Tips: ~The pizza will keep for 2 days refrigerated, after that the semolina starts oxidising and black spots occur. ~Tomato and basil jelly with goat's curd (see recipe Mid meals) is a great salad accompaniment with this pizza! ~High in protein and calcium.

Italian seafood and bean stew

Serves 3 • **Prep** 10 mins • **Cook** 20 mins

1½ cup of fish stock or court bouillon recipe (see Basic recipes)
100ml extra virgin olive oil
120g Desiree potato, peeled and diced small
1 carrot, peeled and finely diced
1 onion small, finely diced
2 cloves garlic
1 tbsp tomato paste
2 tsp thyme
½ can (440g) diced tomatoes
1 can drained and washed cannellini beans
400g white boneless fish (snapper or ocean perch), diced
100g cleaned shelled green prawns
Sea salt and ground white pepper to taste

In a food processor, blend the carrot, onion and garlic until finely chopped. Heat the olive oil in a stainless steel pot, add the carrot, onion and garlic and simmer for 3–4 minutes. Add the tomato paste to the pan, then the crushed tomatoes, thyme and fish stock. Add the potatoes and cannellini beans, cover and simmer until potato is almost cooked.

Add the diced fish and the prawns and cook for 3 minutes or until the fish is cooked through. Drain all liquid and retain in a container. Place the fish soup contents in a food processor and blend until a smooth consistency is achieved. Add a little of the cooking liquor if needed to ensure the puree is the correct thickness and consistency. Add a commercial thickener to the sauce for those on thickened fluids.

Tips: ~The prawns can be omitted and another type of seafood added. ~This is delicious with smoked mussels or clams also. ~To add an extra flavour, serve with a dollop of pea puree in the thick stew (see 'Basic recipes'). ~This is a southern Italian recipe, high in protein, fibre and calcium.

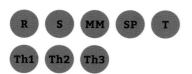

R S MM SP T
Th1 Th2 Th3

Salmon fillet, pease pudding and parsley sauce

Serves 2 • **Prep** 20 mins • **Cook** 15 mins

Salmon
200g salmon fillet, cleaned,
   no blood lines and no skin
   or bones
200ml thickened cream
½ tsp sea salt
¼ tsp ground white pepper
1 egg white
1 pinch nutmeg

Pease pudding
See 'Basic recipes'

Parsley sauce
See 'Basic recipes'

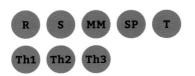

Ensure there are no bones, blood-lines or skin in the salmon, dice and refrigerate. Place the diced salmon, thickened cream, salt and pepper in a food processor and blend for 2 minutes or until it is smooth and mixed together. You may need to stop and scrape down sides of food processor bowl and re-blend slightly to incorporate any lumps that were stuck to the side. Refrigerate the salmon mixture.

Preheat oven to 100°C. Make the pease pudding and start cooking. Pass the salmon mixture through a drum sieve or mouli with smallest holed grating disk (see 'Helpful kitchen equipment').

Refrigerate the salmon mixture. In a clean small stainless steel bowl whisk the egg white with a balloon whisk or a hand mixer until it form peaks (when tipped upside down the whites remain in the bowl). With a metal spoon, carefully fold in the egg white peaks into the chilled salmon mixture.

The salmon mousse is then ready to place into the fish fillet silicon mould (see Contacts and resources for stockists). This mixture will make 4 fish fillets (2 portions). Make the parsley sauce.

Ensure the mould is clean and spray with olive oil spray. Carefully fill each fish indentation with the salmon mousse. Tap to expel any trapped air – a palate knife can be used to scrape away excess mixture from the moulds. Spray the surface of the mould and salmon mousse with olive oil spray. Cover the mould with baking paper.

recipe continues...

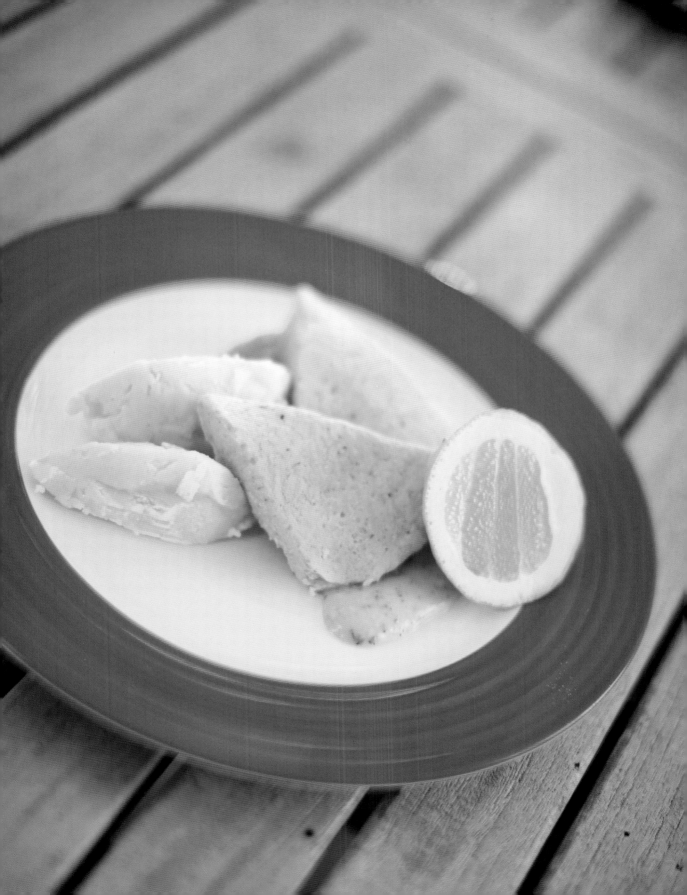

Salmon fillet, pease pudding and parsley sauce

Place in the preheated oven at 100°C for 12 minutes. Meanwhile ensure pease pudding is heated. Remove silicon mould carefully, invert the mould and carefully place the fish on 2 plates and serve with pease pudding and parsley sauce (1-2 tbsp per person) and a wedge of lemon.

Tips: ~If you can't purchase moulds, divide the salmon mousse into four and wrap into 4 sausage shapes using plastic cling wrap. ~Wrap a few more times and twist to tighten the parcels. ~Steam in a bamboo basket or steamer until the fish mousse is cooked (about 10 minutes). ~Other varieties of fish, prawns or lobster work well with this recipe.

Smoked fish brandade

Serves 2 • **Prep** 15 mins • **Cook** 30 mins

250g Desiree potatoes,
   peeled and diced
250g smoked cod
150ml milk
25g butter
1 garlic clove
3 tbsp extra virgin olive oil
2 bay leaves
2 tbsp parsley flakes
Sea salt and pepper to taste

Corn puree
See 'Basic recipes'

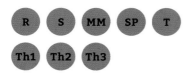

Place potatoes into salted water and simmer for 15-20 minutes or until cooked, drain and leave to dry. Melt butter in a saucepan and sweat off the garlic (no colour) for 1 minute, then add the olive oil, bay leaf and milk.

Flake the fish into the milk, ensuring no bones or skin. Simmer the milk until fish is cooked, then add the parsley flakes. Remove the bay leaves and discard. Make the corn puree.

Drain fish but retain the liquid (this will be used later). Place the fish in a blender and pulse blend until smooth. Place potatoes into a mouli and add the cooking liquor from the fish to the potatoes. Add the smoked cod to the potatoes and pass through the mouli again, season to taste. Serve with the corn puree.

Tips: This can be moulded into shapes or served in ceramic bowl accompanied with corn puree.

Chicken drumstick satay, coconut rice with soy bean puree

Serves 2 • **Prep** 15 mins • **Cook** 20 mins

Chicken drumstick
200g chicken breast (no skin, sinew removed and diced)
200ml thickened cream
1 egg white
½ tsp sea salt
¼ tsp ground white pepper
Olive oil spray

Satay sauce
See 'Basic recipes'

Coconut rice
See 'Basic recipes'

Soy bean puree
See 'Basic recipes'.

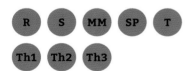

Prepare the satay sauce, by combining all the sauce ingredients and bring to a boil, remove from heat and mix well. If there are any lumps pass through a sieve or use a stick blender.

Ensure there are no bones in the chicken breast, and dice. Place the chicken, thickened cream, salt and pepper in a food processor and blend for 2 minutes or until it is smooth and mixed together. You may need to stop and scrape down sides of food processor bowl and continue to blend to incorporate any lumps stuck to the side. Refrigerate the chicken mixture.

Preheat oven to 100°C. Prepare the soy bean puree and refrigerate. Pass the chicken mixture through a drum sieve or mouli with smallest holed grating disk (see 'Helpful kitchen equipment'). Refrigerate the chicken mixture.

In a clean, small stainless steel bowl whisk the egg white with a balloon whisk or a hand mixer until it forms peaks (when tipped upside down the whites remain in the bowl). With a metal spoon, carefully fold in the egg white peaks into the chilled chicken mixture. The mixture is then ready to place into the chicken drumstick silicon mould (see Contacts and resources for stockists). This mixture will make 6 chicken drumsticks (2 portions).

Ensure the mould is clean and spray with olive oil spray, carefully fill each chicken drumstick indentation. Tap to expel any trapped air, a palate knife can be used to scrape away excess mixture from the moulds.

recipe continues...

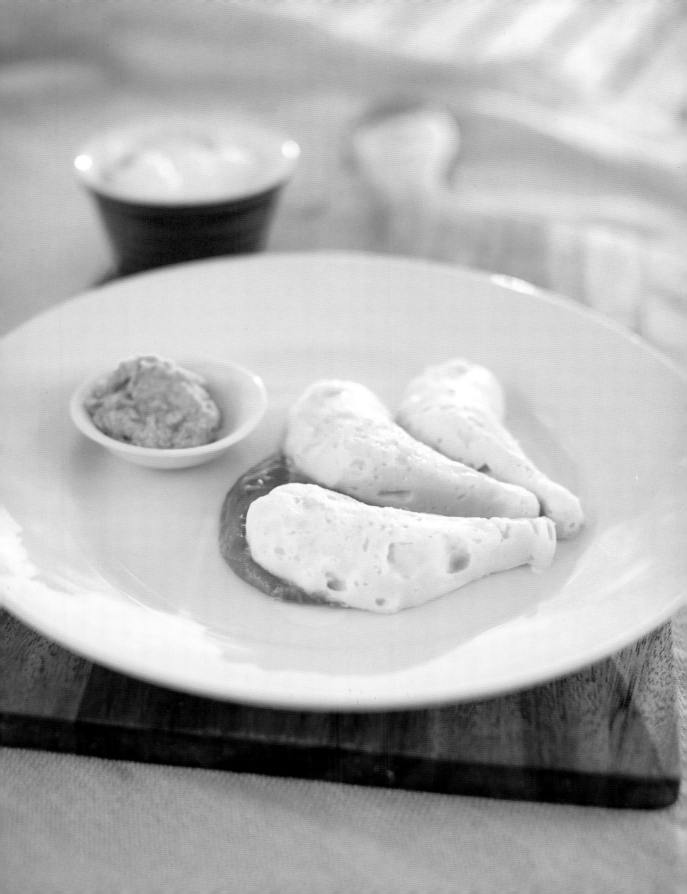

Chicken drumstick satay, coconut rice with soy bean puree

Spray the surface of the mould and chicken stuffing with a little olive oil spray. Cover the mould with baking paper. Prepare the coconut rice.

Place the filled covered silicon mould into a preheated oven at 100°C for 15 minutes, remove and serve immediately. Serve 3 drumsticks with 1-2 tbsp of satay sauce, 1 serve of the coconut rice and 1 serve of the soy bean puree per person.

Tips: ~The chicken does not freeze well but will keep covered in fridge for 48 hours if cooked. It must be reheated delicately by placing on greased baking paper and reheated in a steamer basket (see 'Helpful kitchen equipment'). ~The chicken can also be eaten cold as a salad. ~May also be served with any of the sauces or puree recipes in Basic recipe section, to provide variety. ~If you do not have the chicken moulds, you can use cling wrap to form a nice shape, as follows: divide the mixture into 6 and place each portion into a square of cling wrap; form the chicken into a shape of your choice and wrap, ensuring there are no gaps; wrap in a second lot of cling wrap to ensure a good seal; steam in a steamer basket for 5–8 minutes or until the mixture feels firm to the touch. ~This Asian influenced dish is high in protein.

Story behind the dish: The inspiration for this recipe was to create an Asian-style dish for the new kitchen due to open in 2014 in HammondCare's Braeside Hospital which is located in multicultural south-west Sydney.

Shepherd's pie

Serves 2–3 • **Prep** 15 mins • **Cook** 50 mins

½ tbsp olive oil
300g beef mince
½ onion, finely diced
½ carrot, finely diced
½ celery stick, chopped
1 garlic clove, finely chopped
½ tbsp plain flour
2 tsp tomato paste
50ml red wine
250ml beef stock
1 tbsp Worcestershire sauce
Sprig of thyme
1 bay leaf
1 tsp sea salt
1 pinch pepper

Mash
450g potatoes, chopped
50ml milk
10g butter
50g pecorino cheese,
   finely grated
Freshly grated nutmeg
Parsley oil (optional)
1 tbsp extra virgin olive oil
1 tbsp parsley, finely
   chopped

Pea and mint puree
See 'Basic recipes'

Heat oil in a large saucepan and fry the mince until browned. Put the rest of the oil into the pan, add the vegetables and cook on a gentle heat until soft (about 20 minutes). Add the garlic, flour and tomato paste, increase the heat and cook for 3 minutes, then return the mince to the pan.

Pour over the wine, and boil to reduce it slightly before adding the stock, Worcestershire sauce and herbs. Bring to a simmer and cook, uncovered, for 45 minutes. By this time the sauce should be thick and coating the meat. Check after about 30 minutes – if a lot of liquid remains, increase the heat slightly to reduce the sauce. Season well and then discard the bay leaf and thyme stalks.

While the 'Shepherd's pie' filling is simmering, bring 2 litres of salted water to the boil and cook the potatoes until soft. Remove from heat and drain, add the milk and butter and pass through a potato ricer or mouli. Season to taste and add the cheese.

To assemble the Shepherd's pie, blend the filling in a food processor, return to pan to reduce slightly and season to taste. Divide into two ceramic large ramekins, spoon or pipe the mashed potato on top, cover with foil and heat in oven until centre has reached 75°C (use a digital thermometer).

Remove from oven and discard foil, brush top of cottage pies with parsley oil (1 tbsp extra virgin olive oil stick-blended with 1 tbsp finely chopped parsley, then strain through a sieve).

Serve with pea and mint puree. Can be served also with a small jug of additional gravy. For those on thickened fluids, ensure gravy is the appropriate consistency and any liquid or sauce served is also thickened.

Tips: Any variety of vegetables or mince can be added to this recipe.

Cumberland sausage with bubble and squeak and onion sauce

Serves 2 (makes 6 sausages using sausage silicon moulds)
• **Prep** 20 mins • **Cook** 15 mins

Sausage
200g Cumberland sausages (or good quality British-style pork or beef sausages)
200ml thickened cream
1 tsp thyme, finely chopped
½ tsp sea salt
¼ tsp ground white pepper
½ tbsp flat leaf parsley, finely chopped
1 egg white
Olive oil spray

Bubble and squeak
  See 'Basic recipes'

Onion sauce
  See 'Basic recipes'

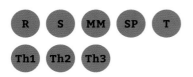

Make onion sauce. Ensure it is blended and passed through a fine sieve. Preheat oven to 100°C. To make the sausages, spray the sausage mould with olive oil spray. Remove the sausage meat from the casing.

Combine all the sausage ingredients (except the egg white) in a food processor and blend until a smooth paste is achieved, this can be then passed through a fine sieve to ensure it is smooth and lump free. Place the sausage puree in the fridge, covered, for 30 minutes.

Meanwhile in a scrupulously clean bowl whisk the egg white until it forms soft peaks. Remove the sausage mix from the fridge and using a stainless steel spoon, carefully fold in the egg whites. Divide the sausage mix into 6 of the greased sausage moulds.

Wipe off any excess filling. Tap the mould to remove any air bubbles. Spray the surface of the sausages in the moulds with olive oil spray and cover with a piece of baking paper. This will stop any crust forming on the sausages.

Make the bubble and squeak and onion sauce (see 'Basic recipes'). Place the sausage moulds in the preheated oven and cook for 15 minutes. Once cooked, carefully remove the mould and invert onto a clean surface allowing the sausages to slide out. Carefully place three sausages per portion onto a hot plate and serve with 2 tbsp of onion sauce and the warm bubble and squeak.

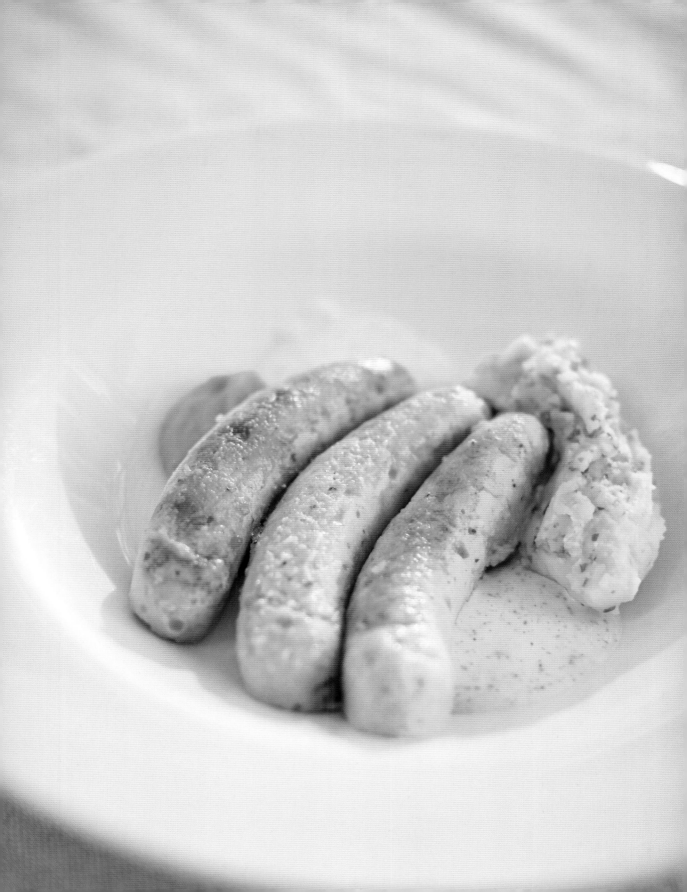

Meatloaf with mushroom sauce and parsnip puree

Serves 2 (Meatloaf recipe yields 4 serves) • **Prep** 12 mins • **Cook** 30–40 mins

Base meat loaf (yields about 1kg)
400g lean beef mince
400g pork mince
200g bacon (with rind removed), finely chopped
1 cup bread crumbs
1 carrot, grated
1 medium onion, finely diced
1 stalk celery, chopped
1 tbsp flat leaf parsley
¼ tsp marjoram
4 tbsp tomato sauce
2 eggs, whisked together
1 tsp Dijon mustard
1 tsp salt
1 tsp ground white pepper
2 tsp Worcestershire sauce
butter to grease the loaf tin

Modified meat loaf
250g cooked meatloaf
80ml beef stock
40ml water
5x small scoops Gelea Instant

Easy pea puree
See 'Basic recipes'

First make the base meat loaf. Mix together both meats, bacon and add salt, pepper and the bread crumbs. Process in a food processor until well combined. Chill the mix. Add the grated carrot and diced onion to the mixture, then add the marjoram, parsley, celery, salt, pepper, Worcestershire sauce, mustard, tomato sauce and the eggs. Mix well. Place in the fridge to cool.

Preheat oven to 180°C. Put the mixture into a greased loaf tin. Smooth the surface and cover with foil. Bake in the centre of the oven for 30 minutes or until the core temperature reaches 75°C. Remove from the oven and allow to cool. When cool, weigh into 250g pieces, retain 1 x 250g piece (this will make 2 portions). All the other pieces of base meat loaf can be wrapped and frozen for a later date.

Blend 250g of the base meat loaf with the beef stock in a food processor, then pass mixture through a mouli or a fine drum sieve with the back of the spoon. This will eliminate any lumps or graininess to the meatloaf. Spoon the Gelea Instant into the water and stir to dissolve. Place the pureed meatloaf into a small non-stick saucepan and add the dissolved Gelea Instant mix. Stir well and bring to boil. Allow to simmer for 2 minutes, continue stirring during this process. Remove from heat.

Pour the hot meat loaf mixture into a small greased individual meat loaf tin or small ramekins (for individual portions). Allow to cool and set. Serve the meatloaf (either warm or cold) with the parsnip puree, easy pea puree and mushroom sauce (see Basic recipes).

Creamed parsnip
See 'Basic recipes'

Mushroom sauce
See 'Basic recipes'

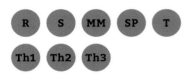

Tips: ~Meatloaf puree can be reheated. ~The easiest way to slice the meatloaf and reheat for a few minutes using a steamer (see Basic recipes). ~Gelea Instant is only able to be reheated to 75°C before it may melt (accurate at the date of printing). So use the thermometer to test the temperature of the sliced meatloaf. ~Gelea Instant is being modified and post-September 2014 the new recipe of Gelea Instant will enable reheating to 100°C (see stockists in 'Contacts and resources' for more information).

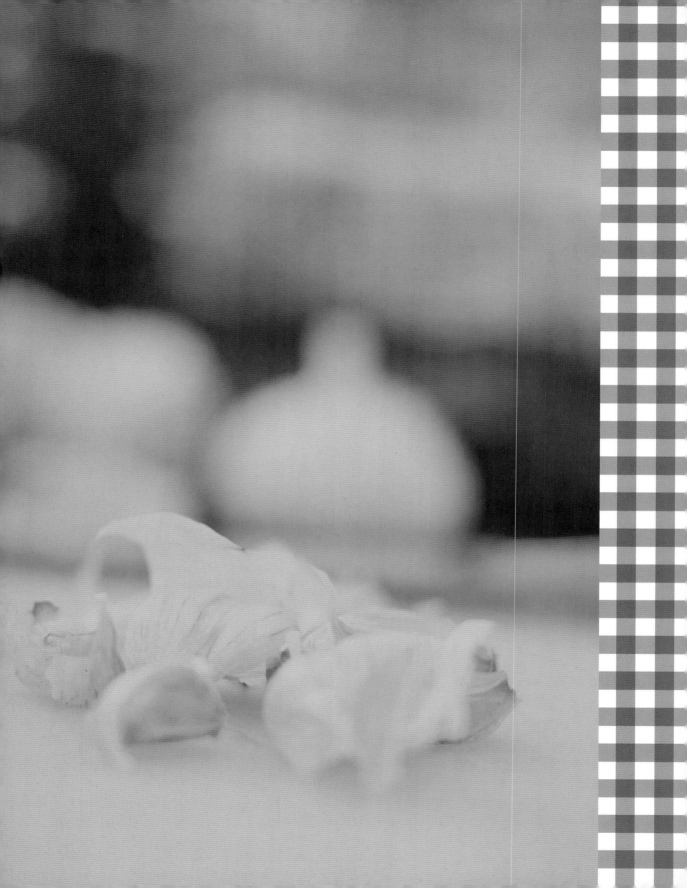

Basic recipes

Basic, but not boring. These recipes form part of many of the dishes featured throughout *Don't give me eggs that bounce* and can also be used in many other creative ways to enhance your favourite meals.

There is also a special section of basic smooth pureed recipes—see the separate introduction for important information for people who require a smooth pureed diet.

Bacon dust

Serves 4 • **Prep** 1 mins • **Cook** 15 mins

4 rashers of rindless bacon,
   thinly sliced

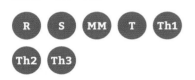

Preheat oven to 190°C and line a tray with baking paper. Lay bacon on tray and bake for 15-20 minutes until crisp and quite dry. Transfer to a paper towel-lined plate and pat dry and free from any grease. Allow to cool. Place bacon in a coffee grinder and process to a fine dust.

Tips: Great flavour enhancer for minced and moist dishes and soups.

Chicken stock

Serves makes 1.5 litres • **Prep** 5 mins • **Cook** 2 hrs

1.8kg chicken carcass
   (cooked or raw)
2 small onions
2 carrots, peeled and
   chopped
1 leek, washed and sliced
1 celery stalk
3 cloves garlic
3 large sprigs of parsley
2 sprigs of thyme
2 bay leaves
1 tsp sea salt
10 black peppercorns
2 litres water

Place all ingredients in a stockpot or any large pot, bring to boil and cook for 2 hours, skimming regularly to remove scum. Strain and use straight away, or allow to cool and place in airtight containers and freeze.

Tips: ~Raw chicken bones make a lighter broth.
~Using a cooked chicken carcass is fine, it will just make it a little darker in colour.

Basic meat stock

Serves makes 1.5 litres • **Prep** 5 mins • **Cook** 4½ hrs

1.5kg meaty bones—veal,
   beef or chicken
Dash of olive oil
2 litres of water
2 carrots, peeled and
   chopped
1 onion, peeled,
4 cloves
1 whole garlic head,
   unpeeled
½ stick of celery, chopped in
   large pieces
½ leek, split and washed
2 bay leaves,
¼ bunch thyme
10 peppercorns
Sea salt

Preheat oven to 220°C. Roast the meat bones in the oven on a tray for 30 mins with a dash of olive oil. Place the roasted bones in a large pot. Add the water, bring to the boil, skimming the liquid to remove the scum. Add more water until it is simmering and no more scum is rising to the surface. Stick the cloves into the onion. Add the rest of the ingredients and simmer slowly for 4 hours. Strain the stock, and allow to cool.

Tips: ~This can be frozen in takeaway containers to use later. ~All dishes taste better using a fresh stock. ~If you are time-poor then choose a good quality ready-made stock.

Court bouillon

Serves makes 750 ml • **Prep** 5 mins • **Cook** 30 mins

750ml water
1 onion, thinly sliced
1 carrot, thinly sliced
½ celery stalk, thinly sliced
2 bay leaves
6 peppercorns
1-2 sprigs of thyme
2 stalks of parsley
3 tsp sea salt
¼ litre dry white wine
   (sauvignon blanc)

Add all the ingredients (except the wine) into a stainless steel pot, simmer for 15 minutes. Add the wine and simmer for 15 minutes more. Strain and discard all the vegetables and aromatics.

Guacamole

Serves 2–4 • **Prep** 5 mins

1 avocado, cut in half, pit
   removed, flesh
   scooped out
1 tbsp sour cream
¼ tsp cumin
1–2 pinches chilli powder
½ tsp sea salt
1 squeeze lime juice
¼ red capsicum, diced
¼ Spanish onion, diced
1 tsp coriander, chopped
½ small tomato seeded and
   finely diced

Remove flesh from the avocado, add lime juice and add all the seasoning. Place the onion and capsicum into a food processor and blend on pulse until finely chopped. Add tomato to the mixture in the food processor and pulse quickly. Remove the mixture from the food processor, drain off any excess juices and add the mixture to the avocado. Add the sour cream and mash all together, adding the chopped coriander at the end.

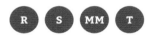

Honey soy sauce

Serves 2-4 • **Prep** 2 mins • **Cook** 1 min

2 tbsp honey
2 tbsp kecap manis (sweet
   soy sauce)
2 tbsp tomato sauce/ketchup
1 tsp lemon juice
Salt and pepper to taste

Combine all ingredients and bring to simmer in a small stainless steel pan for 1 minute. Remove from the heat and serve.

Tips: ~Ideal for a marinade, just don't let it boil.
~For a great chicken marinade, combine all ingredients with a chopped garlic of clove and 1 tsp grated ginger.

Lemon curd

Serves 2–4 • **Prep** 1 min • **Cook** 15 mins

2 whole eggs
2 egg yolks (additional)
200g caster sugar
100g chilled unsalted butter
Zest and juice of 3 lemons

Put the lemon zest and juice, the sugar and the butter into a heatproof bowl. Sit the bowl over a pan of gently simmering water, making sure the water is not touching the bottom of the bowl. Stir the mixture until all the butter has melted.

Lightly whisk the eggs and egg yolk and then stir them into the lemon mixture. Whisk until all of the ingredients are well combined, then leave to cook for 10-13 minutes, stirring every now and again, until the mixture is creamy and thick enough to coat the back of a spoon. It will have reached the right consistency when its temperature reaches 80°C (digital thermometer probe). For a puree, pass through a fine sieve to remove any lumps. If needed, thicken to the desired consistency with a commercial thickener.

Remove the lemon curd from the heat and set aside to cool, stirring occasionally. Once cooled, spoon the lemon curd into sterilised jars and seal. Keep in the fridge until ready to use.

Tips: ~Will keep for 1 week refrigerated and sealed. ~A good addition to French bread and the seedless berry compote. ~Goes well served with chocolate semolina slice, pancakes or alongside puree fruit and custard as an extra flavour.

Macerated strawberries

Serves 1–2 • **Prep** 15 mins

250g punnet strawberries,
   hulled, quartered
2 tbsp Cointreau or fresh
   orange juice
2 tbsp icing sugar, sifted
½ tsp vanilla extract

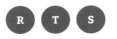

Remove the green tops and cut the strawberries into halves and place in a small bowl. Sprinkle with icing sugar and add the Cointreau or freshly squeezed orange juice and vanilla extract and cover. Leave for 15 minutes to steep. Toss and serve with dessert or with cream and custard.

Tips: ~For a smooth pureed diet, drain the liquid (save it for later use) and puree the strawberries with a stick blender, then pass through a fine sieve to capture all the small seeds.

Mushroom dust

Serves 2–4 • **Prep** 5 mins

50g dried porcini
   mushrooms

Place the dried porcini mushrooms in a coffee grinder and process to a fine dust. Remove any large pieces of mushroom and grind again. Peter says: *'It works best if done in a few small batches.'*

Tips: ~Mushroom dust, like bacon dust, is for flavour encapsulation, a perfect way to add a different flavour dimension to any savoury dish. ~Try it as a flavour enhancer for soups, omelettes or scrambled eggs. ~Keeps well in a sealed container in a cool dry cupboard/pantry.

Mushroom sauce

Serves 4–6 • **Prep** 5 mins • **Cook** 5 mins

50g butter
¼ onion, finely diced
1 clove garlic, finely diced
1 tbsp plain flour
½ cup beef stock
200ml cream
4 button mushrooms, finely diced
1 tbsp mushroom dust (see previous recipe)
Sea salt and pepper to taste

Heat the butter in a small stainless steel pan, add the onion and simmer for 3 minutes (do not allow to burn), then add the garlic and the diced mushrooms, simmer for 1 minute then add the flour, stirring to form a roux.

Heat the stock in the microwave and add to the mushroom and flour roux, stirring to minimise lumps forming. Add the cream, bring to the boil, then simmer for 2 minutes, before adding the mushroom dust. Season to taste.

Tips: ~For a puree, pass through a fine sieve to remove any lumps. ~If needed, thicken to the desired consistency with a commercial thickener.

Onion sauce

Serves 2–4 • **Prep** 5 mins • **Cook** 10 mins

1 tbsp olive oil
2 small Spanish onions, thinly sliced
1 tsp Dijon mustard
2 tbsp balsamic vinegar
300ml beef stock
1 tsp Worcestershire sauce
2 tsp tomato paste
½ tbsp plain flour
Sea salt and ground white pepper

Heat oil in saucepan and add onions, cook until soft but not browned. Add the balsamic vinegar and cook until reduced. Sprinkle onions with the flour, then add the stock, stirring to combine and eliminate any lumps. Add the Dijon mustard, tomato paste and Worcestershire sauce and season to taste.

Tips: ~If the sauce reduces too much, adjust with a little more beef stock. ~The recipe can be processed to make a smooth pureed sauce. ~Place the sauce in a food processor and blend until a smooth, thick sauce is achieved. ~Pass through a fine sieve to remove any lumps of onion.

Parsley sauce

Serves 2–4 • **Prep** 2 mins • **Cook** 5 mins

50g butter
2 tbsp plain flour
½ cup fish stock or chicken
stock (or for a vegetarian
option—court bouillon
recipe or a vegetable
stock).
1 cup thickened cream
2 tbsp flat leaf parsley, finely
chopped
Sea salt and pepper to taste

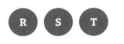

Place butter into a small saucepan and melt, add the flour and stir to form a roux (should resemble breadcrumbs). Cook the roux for 2 minutes, stirring constantly so not allowing it to colour or burn. Heat the stock in the microwave then slowly add it to the roux on a low heat, stir to incorporate the stock and ensure no lumps form. Add the cream and bring to the boil, when the sauce should thicken. Add the parsley and season to taste.

Tips: ~For use as a smooth pureed recipe, blend the sauce with a stick blender and use a commercial thickener to achieve the required consistency. ~If serving parsley sauce with a red meat use chicken stock, if serving with fish use fish stock or for a vegetarian dish use the court bouillon recipe or a vegetable stock. ~Other herbs can be added, such as dill for fish or lemon and thyme for chicken.

Poached chicken breasts

Serves 1– 2 • **Prep** 5 mins • **Cook** 40 mins

1 boneless chicken breast,
  skin off
Water, enough to cover the
  chicken in the saucepan
2 tsp salt
2 tbsp sherry
Piece of fresh ginger
1 clove garlic
Parsley stalks or
  celery leaves

R **T**

Place all ingredients into a small saucepan, add the chicken breast and place on stove. Bring the contents to the boil, turn the chicken breast over and simmer for 3 minutes, before removing the pan from heat. Place a tight fitting lid to the saucepan and leave to cool for 30 minutes in the cooking liquor. Remove the breast and check it is completely cooked through (cut in half horizontally and if it is still pink, simmer for another 2 minutes in the cooking liquor).

Tips: ~Serve cold in a salad, or serve hot. ~To reheat the chicken, the liquid can be reheated and the chicken placed in it until hot enough for serving. ~The cooking liquor can be stored in the fridge and used later for a chicken stock (up to 2 days). ~Store the poached chicken breasts in their liquid, well covered in the fridge, for about 2-3 days. ~Also freeze – either whole, sliced or shredded.

Poached pears

Serves 2–4 • **Prep** 10 mins • **Cook** 20 mins

2 Bosc pears, peeled, cut in
   half and the core removed
3 slices of lemon
500ml water (2 cups)
300g caster sugar (1 cup)
1 bay leaf
Peel from ¼ orange
1 tsp orange juice
1 tsp vanilla essence
1 cinnamon quill
1 pinch nutmeg

Place all ingredients into a saucepan, bring to the boil and turn down to a simmer, ensuring the pears are submerged in the stock syrup (use a side plate as a weight if needed). Simmer for 20 minutes or until the pears are soft (no resistance when a knife is inserted into the flesh). Allow to cool in syrup before serving.

Tips: ~Ideal for all types of fruits—quince, apples, prunes, dried figs and dried apricots. ~Serve with custard (about ½ cup per person) for a simple dessert.

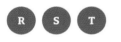

'Select foods and accompaniments that offer variety and contrast, while at the same time avoiding combinations that are awkward or jarring. '

Satay sauce

Serves 2 • **Prep** 15 mins • **Cook** 15 mins

2 tbsp smooth peanut butter
5 tbsp coconut cream
½ tbsp kekap manis (sweet
   soy sauce)
1 tsp cumin
½ tsp sweet chilli sauce

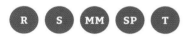

Combine all the ingredients in a saucepan and bring to the boil. Remove from heat and mix well. If any lumps pass through a fine sieve or use a stick blender.

Tips: Recipe can be thickened with a commercial thickener to achieve the required consistency.

Seedless berry compote

Serves 6 • **Prep** 1 min • **Cook** 8 mins

¼ cup caster sugar
300g frozen mixed berries
2 tbsp water

Heat the sugar and 2 tbsp of water in a heavy based saucepan, allow sugar to dissolve down and then bring to boil. Simmer for 3 minutes. Add the berries, allow to come to the boil again and simmer for another 3 minutes. Pour the berry compote into a fine sieve, and using the back of a stainless steel spoon or plastic scraper pass the berry compote through it, leaving all the seeds behind.

Tips: ~The compote can be returned to the stove to reduce further if too runny or can be thickened with a commercial thickener to desired consistency. ~Serve with custard or yoghurt as a light dessert.

Quick gravy

Serves 2 • **Prep** 5 mins • **Cook** 5 mins

1 tbsp red wine
150ml beef stock
   (homemade or bought)
1 tbsp butter
1 tbsp plain flour
1 tsp tomato paste
1 tsp Worcestershire sauce
Sea salt and ground white
   pepper to taste

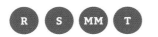

Heat butter in a small saucepan, add the flour and stir until the mixture combines. Add the red wine, stir and allow to evaporate, then slowly add the beef stock, stirring continuously. Add the tomato paste, Worcestershire sauce and season to taste, and simmer for 5 minutes.

Tips: ~If lumps have formed, pass it through a sieve. ~For use as a smooth pureed recipe, pass through a fine sieve and use a commercial thickener to achieve the required consistency. ~This gravy can be the base for other gravies, such as adding sliced mushrooms for a mushroom sauce, adding green peppercorns and 1 tbsp thickened cream for peppercorn sauce. ~For a creamy beef sauce, add 2 tbsp of cream and reduce slightly. ~Other flavour stocks can be used, such as chicken for roast chicken gravy. ~Flavourings can be added such as fresh herbs.

Tomato chutney

Serves 2-4 • **Prep** 10 mins

1 tomato, seeded and diced
100ml tomato sauce recipe
  (see following recipe)
1 pickled onion, sliced finely
1 gherkin, chopped finely
1 tsp gherkin liquid
½ tbsp parsley, chopped
Pinch of cayenne pepper
Salt to taste

Mix all ingredients together in a bowl.

Tips: Goes well with meat and salads.

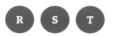

Tomato sauce

Serves 4-6 • **Prep** 5 mins • **Cook** 35 mins

750g ripe tomatoes, chopped
  (or canned diced tomatoes)
1 onion, diced
1 tbsp olive oil
1 garlic clove
1 tsp parsley, chopped
1 tsp basil, chopped
1 tsp thyme, chopped
1 tsp sugar
Sea salt and freshly ground
  pepper to taste

In a large stainless steel pot, fry the onion with the oil (do not allow to brown). Add the remaining ingredients and simmer for 30 minutes or until the tomatoes have been reduced to a thick pulp. Add seasoning to taste. Pass the sauce through a fine sieve using a spatula, to ensure it is smooth. Reduce the sauce further if necessary.

Tips: If needed, thicken with a commercial thickener to the desired consistency.

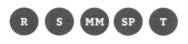

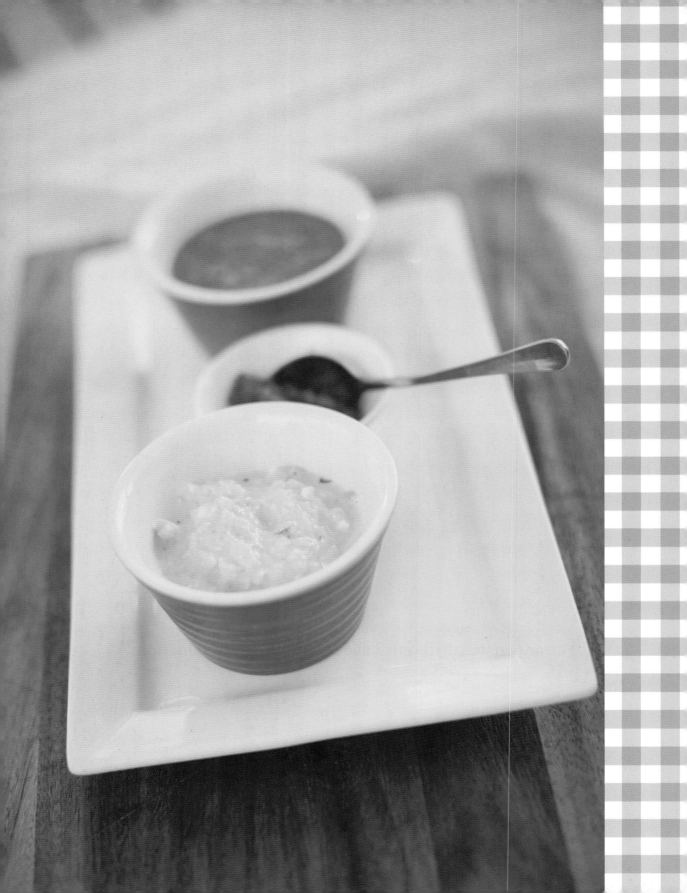

Smooth pureed basics

Many carers and people living with dementia or disability are all too familiar with the challenge of achieving a nutritious, tasty and appetising smooth pureed diet.

Our collection of smooth pureed basics will assist by providing many simple flavour and colour options to enhance mealtimes.

A balanced, smooth pureed meal contains protein (meat, fish, poultry, eggs or legumes), vegetables and carbohydrate (creamed potato, creamed semolina or ground rice). Aim for a third of the plate for each component.

Our pureed recipes can be made and stored in individual portions in the refrigerator for use within 48 hours, making it easier to have a number of accompaniment dishes ready to go at mealtime. Use airtight, freezer-proof containers.

Mix and match different flavour and colour combinations to improve variety. And for convenience, many of these recipes are budget friendly and use basic ingredients including canned legumes and vegetables.

Some, but not all, of the purees in this section can be frozen. Purees with high water content like carrot or starch-based purees, such as potatoes, do not freeze well and can break down when defrosted. The same applies to anything with flour used in the thickening process.

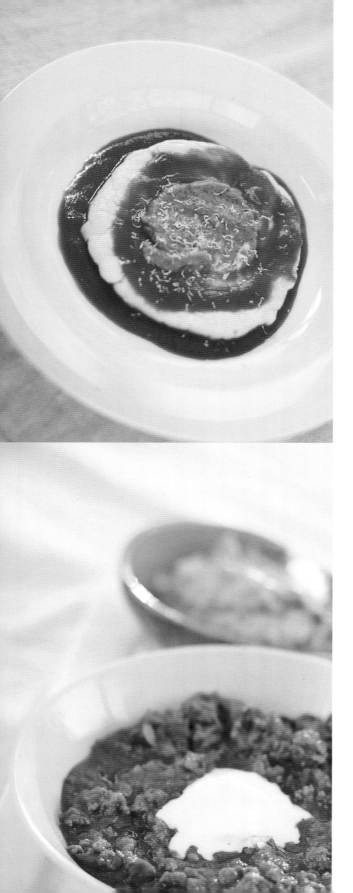

Purees for freezing
- Easy corn puree
- Chickpea puree
- Easy pea puree
- Cannellini bean puree
- Lentil and vegetable puree
- Pease pudding
- Soy bean puree

Carbohydrate purees
Carbohydrates are an important source of energy and should not be forgotten in a smooth pureed diet.

- Coconut rice
- Creamed parsnip
- Creamed potato
- Creamed semolina
- Easy corn puree

Legumes
Legumes are an inexpensive source of protein and fibre. They can be very quick and easy to prepare, straight from the can.

- Chickpea puree
- Easy cannellini bean puree
- Easy pea puree
- Lentil and vegetable
- Pea and mint puree
- Pease pudding
- Refried beans
- Soy bean puree

Vegetables (non starchy)
- Bubble and squeak
- Carrot and orange puree
- Spinach puree

Other
- Guacamole
- Puree mango (moulded)
- Puree pear (moulded)

Bubble and squeak

Serves 2 • **Prep** 10 mins • **Cook** 20 mins

200g peeled Desiree
   potatoes
100g sauerkraut, drained
weight (can be bought
   in a can or a jar)
1 tbsp cream
½ tbsp butter
Sea salt to taste
White pepper to taste
Pinch nutmeg
1 tbsp chopped parsley

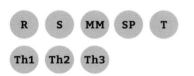

Peel potatoes, cut them into equal pieces and cook in a saucepan with cold salted water. Bring to boil and cook until soft. Drain the sauerkraut and squeeze dry in a clean tea towel—make sure you have 100g. Place the sauerkraut into a food processor and process with the chopped parsley, until smooth. Squeeze any excess water content out of the blended sauerkraut through a fine sieve.

Drain potatoes and return to pan, place on heat and allow to dry out for 2 minutes, add the cream and butter and pass through a mouli (see Helpful kitchen equipment). Add the nutmeg and season to taste with the salt and pepper. Fold in the pureed sauerkraut, reheat in saucepan or microwave (covered on high for 2 minutes).

Tips: Any combination of smooth pureed green vegetable can be added to the mashed potato.

Cannellini bean puree

Serves 2-3 • **Prep** 3 mins

400g cannellini beans,
  drained and rinsed
1 garlic clove
¼ cooked carrot, sliced
2 tbsp olive oil
2 tbsp chopped fresh thyme
Sea salt to taste
Ground white pepper to taste

Drain the cannellini beans and rinse well in running water. Place in food processor with all ingredients and blend until smooth. Season to taste.

Tips: ~Serve hot or cold. ~To heat, place in the microwave for 2 minutes (covered with cling wrap) or heat in a small saucepan.

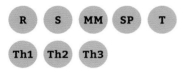

Carrot and orange puree

Serves 2-3 • **Prep** 10 mins • **Cook** 15 mins

200g carrot, peeled
  and thinly sliced
2 tbsp chopped onions
80g Desiree potato,
  peeled and diced
Zest of one orange
1 tbsp butter
Sea salt to taste
Ground white pepper to taste

Cook the potato, carrots and onion in salted water until fully cooked. Drain the water. Grate in zest of orange using a fine grater and add the butter. Pass through a mouli or small drum sieve until smooth. Season with salt and pepper to taste and reheat in saucepan or microwave (covered with cling wrap) for 1 minute.

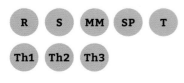

Chickpea puree

Serves 2-4 • **Prep** 5 mins • **Cook** 5 mins

1 x 400g can of chickpeas,
  drained
1 garlic clove, roughly
chopped
Juice of 1 lemon
1/3 cup olive oil
1 tsp ground cumin
1/2 tbsp flat leaf parsley,
chopped finely
Sea salt to taste
Ground white pepper to taste

Wash chickpeas in running water and drain. Combine chickpeas, olive oil, garlic, lemon juice, parsley and cumin in the food processor. Process until smooth. Season with salt and pepper.

Tips: ~Chickpea puree can be served as a dip, or heated warm in microwave or a small saucepan to be served with a main course.

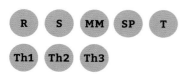

Coconut rice

Serves 2-4 • **Prep** 1 mins • **Cook** 5 mins

1 cup chicken stock
  (or vegetable stock)
5 tbsp coconut cream
6 tbsp rice flour
2 pinches sea salt

Mix 2 tbsp of the cold chicken stock with the rice flour to form a smooth paste/slurry. Bring the rest of the chicken stock to a simmer and with a spoon, stir in the rice flour slurry until it starts to thicken. Add the coconut cream and salt and stir until it slowly thickens to desired consistency (about 4-5 minutes). For a smooth pureed diet, pass the rice through a mouli or blend in the food processor to ensure it is smooth and lump free. Serve immediately.

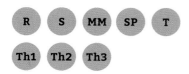

Creamed potato

Serves 2-3 • **Prep** 5 mins • **Cook** 20 mins

250g peeled Desiree
  potatoes
60ml cream
1 tbsp butter
Sea salt to taste
White pepper to taste
Pinch of nutmeg (optional)

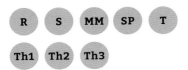

Peel potatoes, cut into equal pieces and cook in pan with salted water.

Drain potatoes and return to pan, place on heat and allow to dry out for 2 minutes. Add the cream and butter to the potatoes and pass through a mouli (see 'Helpful kitchen equipment') or use a potato masher. If using a potato masher the potato mash will need to be passed through a drum sieve to ensure there are no lumps. Season to taste with salt and pepper.

Refried beans

Serves 2-4 • **Prep** 5 mins • **Cook** 10 mins

400g can kidney beans,
  washed and drained
3 tsp ground cumin
1 tsp ground coriander
1 tbsp olive oil
1 clove garlic
1 pinch cayenne pepper
  (optional)
¼ cup water or chicken stock
¼ Spanish onion, finely
  chopped

Heat oil in a saucepan over medium heat. Add onion. Cook, stirring, for 2 minutes or until softened (no colour). Add garlic, cumin, coriander and cayenne pepper, then add the washed beans and cold water or chicken stock. Cook, uncovered, for 5 minutes or until heated through. Remove from heat. Cool slightly. Place beans in food processor and blend until a smooth consistency, a little dash of olive oil can also be added if a little too thick. Season to taste with sea salt.

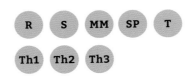

Creamed semolina

Serves 2-4 • **Prep** 1 mins • **Cook** 5 mins

500ml chicken stock
½ cup semolina
1½ tbsp butter
Sea salt to taste
Ground white pepper
  to taste

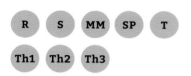

Bring the chicken stock to the boil. Slowly add the semolina until it is all incorporated. Ensure that it is lump free. Add the butter and season to taste.

Serve immediately.

Tips: ~For extra flavour, add grated Parmesan cheese or shaved pecorino. ~Great served as an alternative to mashed potato or to replace a pasta in a smooth pureed diet, minced and moist or a soft diet.

Easy corn puree

Serves 2-3 • **Prep** 3 mins • **Cook** 1 mins

1 x 420g can corn kernels,
  rinsed and drained dry
½ tsp sea salt
¼ tsp ground white pepper
20g melted butter
½ tbsp parsley flakes

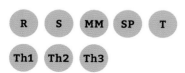

In a food processor, blend the washed and drained corn with melted butter, parsley flakes and seasoning. Continue to blend for another minute or until the corn puree is completely smooth. In the microwave, reheat for 1 minute on high in a microwave-safe container covered with cling wrap, stir and serve.

Easy pea puree

Serves 2-3 • **Prep** 10 mins • **Cook** 20 mins

1 x 420g can of garden
  peas, washed and drained
  (about 260g drained)
½ tsp sea salt
¼ tsp ground white pepper
20g butter, melted
½ tbsp dried parsley flakes

Rinse the peas under cold running water, draining thoroughly. Place peas, melted butter, dried parsley flakes and seasoning into the food processor. Blend on high for one minute, stop and remove the lid and scrape down the sides. Blend for another minute or until the puree is smooth and free from any lumps.

Remove the puree with a scraper and place into a microwavable container. Cover with cling wrap and reheat in the microwave for one minute on high or until the puree is thoroughly heated.

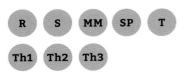

Lentils with vegetables

Serves 2 • **Prep** 20 mins • **Cook** 20 mins

60g red or brown lentils
25g diced carrot
25g diced celery
50g diced potato
20g diced onion
1 pinch of ground cumin
2 tsp white wine vinegar
Sea salt and pepper to taste

Soak the lentils in 400ml of water for 1 hour. Drain the lentils and rinse well. Place in a saucepan and cover with water and cook for 10 minutes. Add the finely diced carrot, celery, onion and potato to the lentils and simmer until cooked (about 25 minutes). Drain and add the cumin and vinegar. Blend with a stick blender, add seasoning to taste and strain through a sieve. For those on thickened fluids, add a commercial thickener to achieve the correct consistency.

Tips: ~Always season dried legumes at the end of the cooking process. ~The salt impacts on the texture of the legumes and can make them hard.

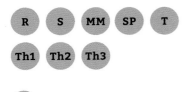

Parsnip puree

Serves 2-4 • **Prep** 10 mins • **Cooking** 15-20 mins

100g Desiree potatoes, peeled
200g parsnip, peeled and cored
2 tbsp butter
Sea salt to taste
Ground white pepper to taste

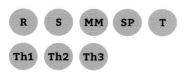

Peel the parsnips and cut in half length wise, cut each half in half again. Carefully remove the hard core from each edge of the quartered parsnip. Chop parsnip strips into equal lengths. Peel potatoes and cut into equal dice, similar size to the parsnips. Place parsnip and potato in salted cold water, bring to the boil and cook until the potato is just cooked (about 15–20 minutes). Drain well.

Place the drained parsnip and potato in a pan and bring to heat to remove any residual moisture, then add the butter and stir through until melted and absorbed. Transfer the parsnip and potato into a mouli and pass through into a clean bowl. Adjust the seasoning with sea salt and ground white pepper.

Pea and mint puree

Serves 2-3 • **Prep** 10 mins • **Cook** 10 mins

about 2 cups
300g frozen peas
1 tbsp chopped onion
2 tbsp butter
1–2 sprigs mint leaves (with stalks)
Sea salt and ground white pepper to taste

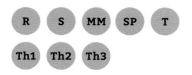

In a saucepan add 1 tsp of the butter and sweat off the onion (no colour). Add the peas and mint (whole sprigs) and cover with salted water, bring to boil and cook for 5 minutes or until peas are tender. Discard the mint sprigs, then drain the peas and onions, but retain the cooking liquid. Add the remaining butter to the peas and about 1- 2 tbsp of the pea cooking liquid. Blend the peas with a stick blender and pass through either a drum sieve using a baker's scraper or a mouli. Season to taste and re-heat in saucepan to serve.

Tips: If the puree is slightly too wet, place in a saucepan under low heat until it reduces to the correct consistency

Pear puree (moulded)

Serves makes 2 half pears • **Prep** 3 mins • **Cook** 2 mins

100g cooked, skinned pear,
  seeds and core removed
  (or use canned pears)
80ml pear juice
½ tsp fresh squeezed
  lemon juice
6 small scoops Gelea
  Instant (see 'Contacts
  and resources')
Olive oil spray

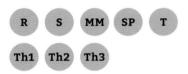

Either poach fresh pears (see 'Basic recipes') or use canned pear slices. Measure 100g of the pear (drained weight) and place in a food processor with the pear juice and the lemon juice. Process until a smooth pureed is produced.

Scrape all the pear puree from the bowl into a small stainless steel saucepan, add the Gelea Instant to the puree pear and stir. Bring the pear to a simmer for 2 minutes, continuously stirring. Remove from the heat, prepare the pear mould (see 'Contacts and resources') by spraying lightly with olive oil spray. Carefully pour the pear puree into the pear indentations in the mould. Place in refrigerator until firm.

Tips: ~Serve with either yoghurt, custard or your choice of dessert. ~For a smooth pureed diet, the pannacotta recipe (see Desserts) is an ideal accompaniment. ~For those on thickened fluids, ensure you serve with double thick custard or Fruche, which is compliant for thickened fluids.

Pease pudding

Serves 2-4 • **Prep** 15 mins • **Cook** 80 mins

½ medium sized onion,
  cut into chunks
1 small carrot, cut into
  4 pieces
1 bay leaf
250g yellow split peas
  (soaked for 1 hour)
1 clove garlic
1 small potato, peeled
  and quartered
25g butter
1 tbsp flat leaf parsley,
  chopped
Sea salt to taste
Ground white pepper to taste

Soak the yellow split peas for 1 hour, then drain them. Place the potato, garlic, onion, carrot, bay leaf and yellow split peas in a saucepan. Cover with cold water and simmer for 1¼ hours. Remove bay leaf and then drain, retaining the cooking liquid. Blend the peas, butter and parsley until smooth and free of lumps. Season to taste and adjust thickness with a little of the cooking liquor until correct texture is reached.

Tips: ~This pudding can be moulded into small Asian tea cups or espresso cups. ~Remove the mini-puddings from the cups when set. ~They can then be reheated in a steamer or on a plate in a microwave, covered, for 2 minutes on high.

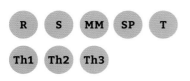

Soy bean puree

Serves 2-4 • **Prep** 5 mins • **Cook** 15 mins

1 cup picked edamame
  beans, shelled (green/
  young soy beans, available
  from Asian grocery stores)
½ cup frozen peas
2 cups water
2 tbsp extra virgin olive oil
1 tsp lemon juice
½ tsp sea salt to taste
¼ tsp ground white pepper
  to taste

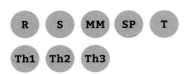

Bring water to boil and place in the shelled edamame beans and simmer for 5 minutes. Add the frozen peas, adding more water if necessary, and simmer until beans and peas are cooked (about 4–5 minutes). Strain the beans and peas, retaining the cooking liquor. Place the beans and peas in a food processor and blend with the oil, lemon juice and seasoning. If too dry, incorporate a little of the cooking liquid. Ensure completely smooth with no lumps. Season to taste, then serve.

Tips: Serve hot or cold. Reheat covered (with cling wrap) in the microwave on high for 1 minute.

Spinach puree

Serves 2-4 • **Prep** 5 mins • **Cook** 5 mins

200g washed baby spinach
1 tbsp flour
50ml thickened cream
100ml milk
½ onion, finely diced
1 tbsp butter
Pinch of grated nutmeg
Sea salt and ground white
  pepper to taste

Place the spinach in a colander and carefully pour boiling water over it until it has wilted. Squeeze the wilted spinach in a clean tea towel until all the moisture has drained out. Chop the spinach roughly with a knife. Place the butter in a saucepan and cook the onions until soft and transparent (no colour). Add the flour and stir for 2 minutes, then add the milk and cream, stirring continuously until the sauce has thickened. Remove from heat and place the sauce and spinach in a food processor and blend until a smooth pureed is formed, season with nutmeg and salt and pepper to taste.

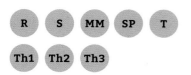

Tips: ~Serve hot or cold. If consistency is too wet, further reduce in a saucepan, or thicken with a commercial thickening agent. ~If overcooked, the lovely green colour will turn brown!

Mango puree (moulded)

Serves 2 x 50g • **Prep** 2 mins • **Chilling** 45 mins

1 ripe mango
1 tsp lime juice
6 small scoops Gelea Instant
  (see specialised suppliers)
Olive oil spray

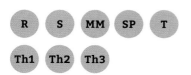

Remove all the flesh from the mango, discard the skin and seed, and process flesh in a food processor until smooth. Measure out 200ml of mango puree (if a little less top up with water to make up the volume to 200ml) and place in a mixing bowl. Add the lime juice and then stir in the Gelea Instant and ensure it is mixed into the mango pulp.

Place the puree into a small stainless steel saucepan and bring to simmer, stirring continuously. Allow to simmer for 2 minutes. Remove from heat. Lightly grease a mould (either a melon mould or a sliced meat plastic mould) with olive oil spray. Pour the warm mango puree into two of the indentations and allow to set in the refrigerator for about 45 minutes.

Tips: ~Try this recipe with other types of fruit also— let your imagination run wild. ~If you use fruit that has fibrous bits, strain the puree through a fine sieve before you add the lime juice and Gelea Instant.

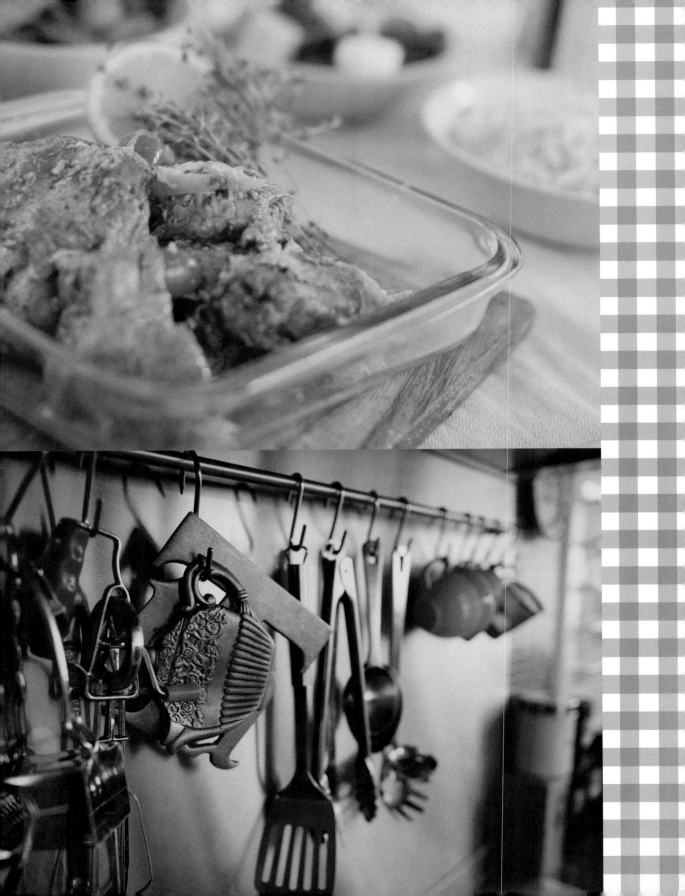

Meal plans

Recipes in *Don't give me eggs that bounce* are designed
to be part of day-to-day eating, as well as providing
hero dishes for special occasions.

To assist with daily food planning, the following meal plans
cover texture options seen throughout the book—regular,
soft, minced and moist and smooth pureed. There are also
plans for small serves and finger foods.

Some people with advancing dementia will not be able
to eat the volume of food we have included and so portion sizes
can be adjusted if needed. If someone has a poor appetite
and is losing weight, prioritise the meat, dairy and richer,
creamier foods that the person enjoys to maximise
calorie and protein intake.

For all meal plans, it is important to remember that fluids
must be thickened for people with this dietary recommendation.
Some dishes will also need to be thickened such as thinner
soups, sauces and smoothies. As a reminder you'll see
Th where thickening may be needed.

Regular texture

Breakfast	Perfect boiled egg, sourdough soldiers Tea or coffee Th Water or juice Th
Morning tea	Fruit salad with vanilla honey yoghurt Th Tea or coffee Th
Lunch	Reuben sandwich (corned beef and cheese toasted sandwich) Water Th
Afternoon tea	Strawberry almond milkshake Th
Dinner	Slow cooked lamb shoulder, baked potato, carrots and green beans Lemon ricotta cake with yoghurt and ricotta Water Th

Small serves

Some people who have very small appetites will require small and frequent meals. The goal is to maximise the nutritional value of everything they eat. As above, fluids must be thickened for those who require it—see Th.

Breakfast	Ricotta and prune pot Small banana Tea or coffee Th Water Th
Morning tea	Peach, berry and oatmeal smoothie Th
Lunch	Small serve Mushroom and ham frittata, one piece mix grain bread and small salad of three cherry tomato and 3 slices cucumber Water Th
Afternoon tea	Small piece of cheese (20g) and 4 wholemeal, savoury biscuits Tea or coffee Th
Dinner	Small serve Pan fried ocean trout, potato cake and peas Small serve Impossible pie with custard and macerated strawberries
Supper	Banana and raspberry muffin Tea or coffee Th

Finger food

The finger food meal plan is very high in energy as often those requiring finger food are more active. As above, thicken fluids or dishes as required—see Th.

Breakfast	Leg ham and Gruyere and spinach croque monsieur, cut into quarters Tea or coffee Th Water or juice Th
Morning tea	Chocolate and peanut smoothie Th
Lunch	Hearty ploughman's lunch (egg, cheese, ham, salad vegetables cut into chunks and bread) Water Th
Afternoon tea	Banana loaf cake Tea or coffee Th
Dinner	Pea and salmon fishcakes with tartare sauce and boiled potato Raw fruit pudding Water Th
Supper	Chocolate semolina slice

Soft foods

Breakfast	Bircher Muesli Tea or coffee Th Water Th
Morning tea	Chocolate and peanut smoothie Th
Lunch	Spanish omelette with wilted spinach Water Th
Afternoon tea	French toast with mashed banana Tea or coffee Th
Dinner	Italian sausage, cannellini bean casserole with tomato Soft brown bread Strawberry Eton mess Water Th
Supper	½ cup milk to drink Th

Minced and moist

Breakfast	Pear and Fruche Tea or coffee Th Water Th
Morning tea	Mango smoothie Th
Lunch	Lentil soup with crumbled sausage and soaked bread Water Th
Afternoon tea	Cheese and tomato custard Tea or coffee Th
Dinner	Beef, shiraz and mushroom casserole with creamed potato and pea puree Irish rice pudding with macerated sultanas Water Th
Supper	½ cup milk to drink Th

Smooth pureed

Breakfast	Classic scrambled eggs Soaked brown bread Tea or coffee Th Water Th
Morning tea	High protein milkshake Th
Lunch	Pease pudding with spinach puree Water Th
Afternoon tea	Tomato jelly, basil pesto and goat's curd Tea or coffee Th
Dinner	Italian seafood and bean stew with potato Vanilla pannacotta with puree pear
Supper	½ cup milk to drink Th

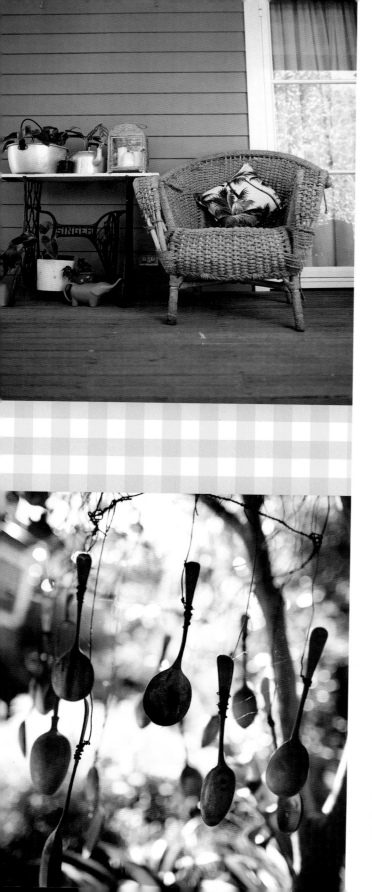

Meal plan nutritional details

The nutritional goals for each recipe have been based on the work done for the Queensland Meals on Wheels Nutrition Manual[5].

Goals for meals across the day and meal plans were based on a minimum 76kg reference male at 126kJ/kg/day = 9.6MJ, 1.2g protein/kg/day = 91.2g. Recipes included in this book are high in energy and protein as dietary restrictions are not warranted unless specifically recommended by a health professional for individuals.

Main meals (lunch and dinner) provide at least 1800kJ of energy and 25g of protein when served with recommended side dishes. Note that sausage recipes have been included for popularity, however high quality sausages should be used to ensure at least 20g protein per serve is provided.

Lighter meals including breakfasts provide at least 1200kJ and 10g protein per serve, with some being nutritionally equivalent to a lunch or dinner meal. Desserts all provide at least 1500kJ and 5g protein. Mid meals are all at least 600kJ (most >1000kJ) and contain at least 5g of protein. A number of the desserts and mid meals also are high calcium, containing at least 200mg calcium. A small serve would be about two thirds of a normal serve and this is what we have used in the meal plan for small serves.

People on a low salt diet for medical reasons should follow the recommendations of doctor or health professionals in choice and preparation of food.

Contacts and resources

Information in this section covers helpful contacts and resources in Australia but similar stockists, support organisations and food suppliers will be available in most countries. HammondCare's Dementia Centre operates internationally.

Commercial thickener information

When thickening fluids for people with dysphagia, it is important that recipes are tried and tested to ensure they are not placing a person at risk of aspiration.

The most commonly used thickeners are listed below. Although the recipes in this book have been formulated with particular products, we do not necessarily endorse that product and each person should decide for themselves which product they prefer. However, when following recipes, you will need to pay particular attention to the amounts of powder and modify quantities according to the product you have purchased.

Further retailers for thickening agents, who sell products to individuals (rather than companies, such as hospitals and nursing homes) may be found on the Internet. It is recommended that you complete your own research where possible to find competitive pricing. Remember, those who are part of the Department of Veterans' Affairs may be eligible for subsidised products.

Flavour Creations: Instant thick powder and pre-thickened fluids

Stockists of Flavour Creations for each Australian state and territory can be found by visiting www.flavourcreations.com.au and clicking on the 'where to buy' page or by phoning head office on 07 3373 3000.

Nestle: Resource ThickenUp Clear powder

Stockists for ThickenUp Clear for each Australian state and territory can be found by visiting www.nestlehealthscience.com.au and clicking on 'products' and then 'stockists' or by phoning 1800 025 361 or 1800 671 628.

Gelea and Spuma Instant

Gelea Instant and Spuma Instant are available from Biozoon Food Innovations, part of Prestige Products Group Pty Ltd. Visit www.molecular-gastronomy.com.au, phone 1300 652 198 or email sales@prestigeproducts.com.au

Online food suppliers

Aussie Farmers Direct
www.aussiefarmers.com.au or phone 1300 645 562 (8am–8pm Monday to Friday, 8:30am–5pm Saturday AEDST).

Coles online
www.shop.coles.com.au or phone 1800 455 400 (Monday to Friday, 6am–midnight, Saturday 7am–10pm and Sunday 8am–6pm AEDT).

Woolworths online

www2.woolworthsonline.com.au or phone 1800 000 610 (Monday to Friday, 6am–10pm, Saturday 6am–10pm, Sunday 8am–6pm)

Food moulds

Puree Food Molds

Online ordering system at www.pureefoodmolds.com or email info@pureemolds.com

Prestige products

www.molecular-gastronomy.com.au or phone 1300 652 198.

Home delivered meals

Meals on Wheels

For your local provider phone the Meals on Wheels Association on 02 8219 4200 or visit www.mealsonwheels.org.au

Tender Loving Cuisine (TLC)

Provides meal delivery to homes in Sydney, Melbourne and south-east Queensland. Phone 1800 801 200 or 02 9713 5355 or visit www.tlc.org.au

Gourmet Dinner Service

Provides fresh cooked meals to homes in Sydney, Brisbane, Melbourne, Canberra and coastal areas of NSW and Queensland. Phone 1300 131 070 or visit www.gourmetdinnerservice.com.au

Choice Fresh Meals

Fresh cooked meals delivered to homes in Melbourne, Mornington Peninsula, Geelong and Bellarine Peninsula. Phone 1300 430 488 or visit www.choicefreshmeals.com.au

Eat@home

Fresh cooked meals delivered to homes in Melbourne, Mornington Peninsula and Geelong. Phone 1300 855 722 or visit www.eatathome.com.au

Manor Meals

Fresh cooked meals delivered to homes in the Melbourne area. Phone 03 5977 6966 or visit www.snrs.com.au/services/home-delivered-meals/

Home Chef

Freshly cooked meals served frozen in the Perth area. Phone 08 9378 2544 or visit www.homechef.com.au

Cuisine Courier

Many takeaway restaurants will home deliver meals. Contact your local Cuisine Courier for restaurants in your area that will home deliver meals. Phone 1300 678 933 or visit www.cuisinecourier.com.au

Dementia-related support organisations

The Dementia Centre

The Dementia Centre, part of HammondCare, works to empower everyone from health professionals and managers to carers in the home to take action to improve quality of life for people living with dementia. Our service offers evidence-based practice advice drawn from extensive and ongoing research programs, backed by experience in the field. The Dementia Centre provides services to people living across Australia and internationally.

Phone +61 2 8437 7355 or visit www.dementiacentre.com.au Address: Dementia Centre, Pallister House, Greenwich Hospital, 97-115 River Road Greenwich, NSW 2065 Australia.

Dementia Behaviour Management Advisory Services (DBMAS)

The DBMAS program is an Australian Government initiative which provides clinical support for people caring for someone with dementia who is demonstrating behavioural and psychological symptoms of dementia (BPSD) which are impacting on their care. It provides a 24 hour a day helpline as well as face to face visits.

Phone 1800 699 799 or
visit www.dbmas.org.au

Alzheimer's Australia

Alzheimer's Australia provides information and education on dementia and runs programs and services such as counselling and support groups.

Phone 1800 100 500 or visit www.
fightdementia.org.au

My Aged Care

My Aged Care is a service run by the Australian Government Department of Social Services that provides useful information and advice on all areas of aged care, including community care, nursing homes, staying at home and staying healthy.

Phone 1800 200 422 (8am–8pm Monday to Friday, 10am–2pm Saturday)
or visit www.myagedcare.gov.au

Commonwealth Respite and Carelink Centres

Commonwealth Respite and Carelink Centres are information centres for older people, people with disabilities and those who provide care and services. They provide free and confidential information on community aged care, disability and other support services available. They can also provide you with information about the Assisted Shopping program.

Phone 1800 052 222 or
visit www9.health.gov.au/ccsd

Independent Living Centre

The Independent Living Centre is a service, staffed by occupational therapists, that provides independent and impartial information and advice about equipment (such as adaptive cutlery, special cups), assistive technologies and home modifications. They do not sell equipment but can provide advice about suitable and available products and where to purchase them.

Each state and territory has an Independent Living Centre. For NSW, QLD, Victoria, SA, WA, Tasmania and NT a toll-free helpline will automatically transfer to the appropriate centre—phone 1300 885 886. ACT residents should phone 02 6205 1900. The national website is www.ilcaustralia.org

Eating, drinking support organisations

Speech Pathology Australia

Speech Pathology Australia can provide information about speech pathology services and help locate local speech pathologists. Phone 1300 368 835 or visit www. speechpathologyaustralia.org.au

Dietitians Association of Australia

Dietitians Association of Australia provides general information about food and diet and can help locate local dietitians. Phone1800 812 942 or visit www.daa.asn.au

Occupational Therapy Australia

Occupational Therapy Australia supports the work of occupational therapists and can assist in finding an occupational therapist in your area. Phone 1300 682 878 or visit www.otaus.com.au

Helpful kitchen equipment

Food processor

Repetitive tasks in the preparation of food are made easier with a food processor. The term usually refers to an electric appliance, although there are some manual devices. Food processors are similar to blenders with the main difference being food processors use interchangeable blades and disks instead of a fixed blade. Also, their bowls are wider and shorter, in keeping with the solid and semi-solid foods prepared in a food processor. Usually little or no liquid is required in the operation of the food processor, unlike a blender, which requires some liquid to move the food around the blade.

Stick blender

Blending ingredients or pureed food in the container in which they are being prepared is one advantage of a stick blender. They may be used for pureeing soups and emulsifying sauces. Some can be used while a pan is on the stove.

Mouli grater

A mouli grater is hand-operated kitchen utensil designed for pureeing small quantities of food. The device consists of a small metal drum with holes that grate the food and a handle for turning the drum.

Coffee grinder

A coffee grinder uses blades rotating at high speed and can be either specifically for coffee and spices, or a general-use home blender. Blade grinders create 'dust' that can be used in cooking, such as ground dried mushrooms to make a mushroom dust. They are reasonably priced and are great for grinding almost anything including nuts, popcorn and of course, coffee—let your imagination run riot!

Cream whipper

A cream whipper is a steel cylinder or cartridge filled with nitrous oxide (N2O) that is used as a whipping agent in a whipped cream dispenser. The nitrous oxide in whipped cream chargers is also used in molecular gastronomy for making hot and cold foams and is ideal for making smoothies and dessert mousses. Several recipes in *Don't give me eggs that bounce* highlight how to make great texture-modified desserts and beverages using this process.

Digital scale

Access to a finely calibrated scale that can measure ingredients accurately is vital and is one advantage of digital scales. Older-style mechanical scales are quite inaccurate for small amounts. Ideally your scales will have a 1g increment which will enable greater precision, particularly when using thickeners.

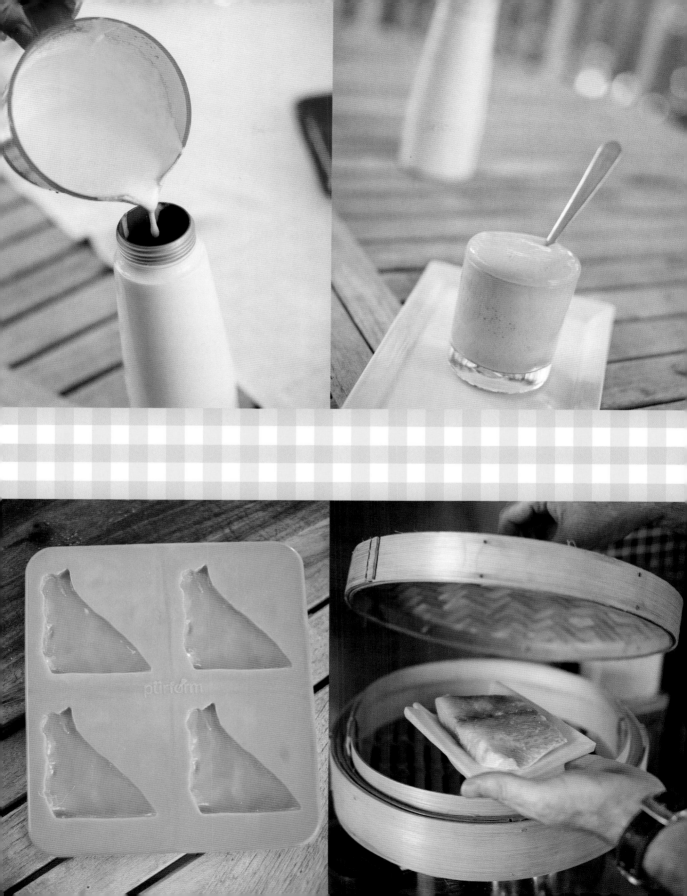

Silicon moulds

When preparing pureed meals, it is great to experiment using silicon moulds to 'shape the food'. There are a variety of silicon moulds available in pastry shops (cookie and muffin moulds) which can be used to improve a person's dining experience and dignity. There are also specialised moulds that are manufactured to assist people with dysphagia (see 'Contacts and resources').

Digital probe

A digital probe is essential for measuring accurate core temperatures of food. It is a requirement in Australia in aged care and hospitals (at time of publishing) that core temperatures of high-risk foods reach 75°C. The probe removes the guess work. In various recipes in *Don't give me eggs that bounce* core temperatures are listed for cooking processes. An oven thermometer is also recommended (leave in oven so temperature can be seen through the glass).

Other equipment

Other common kitchen equipment that will be helpful in the preparation of food, drinks and dishes from *Don't give me eggs that bounce* include:

Slow cooker—ideal for cooking casseroles and a great way to have the aroma of cooking wafting from the kitchen.

Baker's scraper/pastry scraper—essential for passing purees through a drum sieve and can be either plastic or metal.

Bamboo or aluminium steamer baskets with lid—ideal for steaming vegetables, fish or chicken or reheating or cooking moulded foods. See how to use a steamer in 'Basic recipes'. They are not suitable for Hazard Analysis Critical Control Point (HACCP) kitchens and aged care or hospital kitchens catering for vulnerable people.

High-temperature rubber spatula—can be used for cooking, passing purees through a sieve and for scraping foods from bowls.

Ovenproof ramekins—great for desserts, custards and soufflés. A necessity for a modified diet.

Measuring jugs, cups and spoons—all our recipes stipulate weight, cups or spoons. Also see our 'Conversions' section.

Balloon whisk—essential for incorporating air into desserts and whipping cream.

Muslin cloth—handy for passing liquids in a sieve to filter out any sediment. Ideal for passing stocks and also the court bouillon recipe. It can be used also for wrapping roulades, which can then be poached while retaining their shape and integrity.

Sieves—The conical sieve is essential for straining stocks, sauces, passing mousses. When purchasing, look for a fine conical sieve, particularly important for preparing modified meals and purees. The second is a drum sieve which are ideal for passing through meat purees using a baker's spatula.

References

Introduction—
A few words about dementia

1. Alzheimer's Disease International (2011) World Alzheimer Report 2011: The Benefits of Early Diagnosis and Intervention, Alzheimer's Disease International, London http://www.alz.co.uk/world-report-2011

Chapter 2

2. Dietitians Association of Australia. DAA Evidence based practice guidelines for the nutritional management of malnutrition in adult patients across the continuum of care. Nutrition & Dietetics Journal 2009; 66: S1-S34. http://onlinelibrary.wiley.com/doi/10.1111/ndi.2009.66.issue-s3/issuetoc Accessed 13 November 2012

3. Rist G, Miles G, Karimi L. The presence of malnutrition in community-living older adults receiving home nursing services. Nutrition & Dietetics 2012; 69: 46–50

Chapter 3

4. The key reference for this chapter is: Dietitians Association of Australia and The Speech Pathology Association of Australia Limited (2007). Texture-modified food and thickened fluids as used for individuals with dysphagia: Australian standardised labels and definitions. Nutrition & Dietetics 64 (Suppl.2): 553-576.

Meal plans

5. Meals on Wheels Nutrition Manual: Nutrition guidelines for the provision of home delivered meals. Angela Malberg 2012. Queensland Meals on Wheels Association Inc. Strathpine Centre, QLD 4500 Australia

Nutritional information

Recipe Name	Energy	Energy
Banana and coconut porridge	1748kJ	418 cal
Bircher muesli modified	2441kJ	583 cal
Bircher muesli	1780kJ	425 cal
Classic scrambled eggs	2552kJ	610 cal
Honey and banana Weetbix	3046kJ	728 cal
Israeli shakshuka	1477kJ	353 cal
Leg ham and gruyere and spinach croque monsieur	3933kJ	939 cal
Pear with yoghurt	1557kJ	372 cal
Perfect boiled egg with sourdough soldiers	1726kJ	412 cal
Baked ricotta and prune pot	1215kJ	290 cal
Ricotta hot cakes with banana and vanilla honey	1982kJ	473 cal
Toasted muesli	2063kJ	493 cal
Banana and raspberry muffins	2453kJ	586 cal
Banana loaf cake	2193kJ	524 cal
Berowra ginger bread	1796kJ	429 cal
Carrot, sultana and walnut cupcake	1327kJ	317 cal
Cheese and tomato custards	1894kJ	453 cal
Chocolate and peanut butter smoothie	1169kJ	279 cal
Chocolate semolina 'fudge'	1046kJ	250 cal
French toast	1097kJ	262 cal
Fruit salad with vanilla honey yoghurt	1189kJ	284 cal
High protein milkshake	974kJ	233 cal

Protein	Total fat	Carbo-hydrate	Dietary fibre	Calcium	Iron
10.3g	24.6g	38.0g	5.4g	209.2mg	1.3mg
15.9g	12.9g	94.6g	11.1g	259.6mg	0.0mg
12.7g	10.3g	66.2g	6.9g	296.9mg	2.2mg
22.7g	46.0g	26.5g	1.5g	133.8mg	2.8mg
11.7g	51.6g	54.9g	4.8g	216.5mg	4.1mg
16.4g	14.2g	36.7g	5.6g	126.1mg	3.6mg
56.3g	62.4g	37.3g	3.5g	1059.9mg	4.9mg
13.8g	7.1g	59.2g	6.0g	442.1mg	0.6mg
21.3g	24.8g	25.5g	1.5g	97.5mg	2.8mg
11.1g	19.3g	18.3g	2.0g	164.8mg	1.0mg
18.6g	16.5g	62.5g	3.2g	316.5mg	1.6mg
7.1g	29.5g	48.5g	6.9g	53.4mg	3.3mg
12.1g	39.2g	44.6g	6.8g	136.1mg	2.1mg
9.6g	36.2g	40.0g	4.6g	89.3mg	1.6mg
5.9g	13.6g	71.8g	2.5g	196.7mg	2.4mg
7.6g	24.7g	15.9g	3.5g	70.2mg	1.5mg
32.7g	28.1g	17.9g	0.7g	679.1mg	1.2mg
9.6g	11.7g	34.0g	1.3g	193.1mg	0.3mg
5.8g	7.9g	39.4g	1.2g	102.2mg	1.1mg
11.7g	10.4g	30.4g	1.9g	105.0mg	1.3mg
10.1g	5.9g	43.3g	6.5g	269.2mg	1.1mg
11.9g	7.8g	29.6g	0.9g	354.0mg	0.2mg

Recipe Name	Energy	Energy
Mango smoothie	680kJ	162 cal
Peach, coconut and banana oatmeal smoothies	1033kJ	247 cal
Pete's arancini	1203kJ	288 cal
Raw fruit pudding, coconut icing	1467kj	350 cal
Scones	2025kJ	484 cal
Strawberry almond milkshake	821kJ	196 cal
Tomato jelly, basil and goats curd	1131kJ	270 cal
Vanilla and yoghurt ice cream	845kJ	202 cal
Pikelets, jam and cream	1862kJ	445 cal
Welsh rare-bit	1996kJ	477 cal
Bacon and lentil soup with crusty sourdough bread	2068kJ	494 cal
Ham and mushroom frittata	2350kJ	561 cal
Meat loaf with simple tomato chutney	1622kJ	387 cal
Hearty ploughman's lunch	2846kJ	680 cal
Home made pizza	3247kJ	776 cal
Pea and salmon fishcakes with tartare sauce	2781kJ	664 cal
Reuben sandwich with sauerkraut	2972kJ	710 cal
Duck Sausage with braised lentils	3114kJ	744 cal
Pan fried ocean trout, potato cake and pea puree	3227kJ	771 cal
Pickled pork neck, red cabbage and mustard sauce	2256kJ	539 cal
Roast chicken breast, cannellini bean puree, roasted tomatoes	2459kJ	587 cal
Semolina gnocchi with tomato and olive stew	3993kJ	954 cal
Slow braised beef cheeks with parsnip puree	1849kJ	442 cal
Janni's slow cooked shoulder of lamb	1863kJ	445 cal

Protein	Total fat	Carbo-hydrate	Dietary fibre	Calcium	Iron
6.8g	5.1g	21.2g	1.5g	190.6mg	0.3mg
9.1g	11.4g	25.2g	2.2g	225.2mg	0.9mg
10.5g	12.4g	32.8g	1.1g	94.6mg	0.7mg
5.3g	13.5g	49.1g	8.5g	80.2mg	2.8mg
6.3g	24.5g	60.1g	2.1g	106.0mg	0.6mg
8.4g	10.8g	15.5g	1.6g	221.2mg	0.7mg
12.2g	18.6g	10.5g	6.0g	147.2mg	2.3mg
6.4g	9.5g	22.1g	2.0g	0.0mg	0.0mg
11.5g	20.8g	52.9g	1.9g	163.2mg	0.7mg
18.8g	36.3g	17.3g	1.6g	428.4mg	1.3mg
31.0g	18.5g	46.4g	11.6g	202.9mg	5.9mg
45.2g	41.7g	1.8g	0.8g	373.9mg	2.4mg
33.9g	13.4g	30.5g	4.0g	78.2mg	3.7mg
25.4g	37.9g	55.3g	6.9g	329.2mg	3.1mg
35.0g	40.3g	65.7g	4.9g	491.3mg	3.2mg
31.8g	36.4g	49.9g	5.5g	69.3mg	3.3mg
41.1g	40.7g	41.2g	8.2g	539.0mg	6.2mg
41.8g	37.2g	56.3g	9.3g	119.0mg	7.3mg
48.2g	47.0g	33.8g	10.9g	412.4mg	4.5mg
44.9g	23.3g	33.3g	7.2g	87.2mg	2.7mg
32.0g	40.5g	21.4g	9.1g	116.8mg	3.2mg
28.2g	66.0g	59.9g	7.3g	654.8mg	2.8mg
37.5g	24.7g	14.1g	7.4g	90.5mg	5.1mg
51.7g	25.5g	1.2g	1.9g	28.7mg	5.4mg

Recipe Name	Energy	Energy
Cherry jelly cheese cake	2292kJ	548 cal
Impossible pie with macerated strawberries	1867kJ	446 cal
Irish rice pudding with sultanas	2341kJ	559 cal
Lemon ricotta cake	1577kJ	377 cal
Rich chocolate mousse	3712kJ	887 cal
Strawberry Eton mess	1786kJ	427 cal
Vanilla pannacotta	1855kJ	443 cal
Blood orange foam	342kJ	82 cal
Green vegetable cocktail	970kJ	232 cal
Grilled grapefruit and cherry foam	307kJ	73 cal
Lemonade	338kJ	81 cal
Watermelon, lime and mint foam	228kJ	54 cal
Cottage pie	2332kJ	557 cal
Italian sausage	1967kJ	470 cal
Risoni with bolognaise sauce	3289kJ	786 cal
Spanish omelette with wilted spinach	2216kJ	529 cal
Steamed barramundi with ratatouille	3522kJ	841 cal
Beef, Shiraz and mushroom casserole	2646kJ	632 cal
Boston baked beans, scrambled egg and bacon dust	2376kJ	568 cal
Chilli con carne	2450kJ	585 cal
Lentil soup with crumbled sausage	2574kJ	615 cal
Moroccan lamb, sultanas and green olives	2647kJ	632 cal
Pizza soufflé	2828kJ	676 cal
Seafood chowder	2203kJ	526 cal

Protein	Total fat	Carbo-hydrate	Dietary fibre	Calcium	Iron
9.9g	33.1g	54.2g	1.6g	0.0mg	0.0mg
9.1g	24.2g	49.3g	2.2g	160.6mg	0.8mg
8.1g	32.4g	60.7g	1.3g	183.1mg	0.8mg
11.4g	16.7g	45.4g	1.6g	256.4mg	1.0mg
6.6g	65.6g	72.0g	1.0g	95.6mg	3.0mg
5.6g	20.3g	57.6g	1.2g	108.0mg	0.6mg
6.5g	36.9g	23.6g	0.0g	154.6mg	0.0mg
1.0g	0.2g	17.3g	2.4g	0.0mg	0.0mg
2.9g	13.0g	24.6g	3.7g	55.8mg	2.1mg
0.9g	0.2g	15.6g	2.2g	0.0mg	0.0mg
0.4g	0.1g	19.5g	0.5g	22.3mg	0.4mg
0.8g	0.5g	10.9g	2.3g	0.0mg	0.0mg
30.5g	34.9g	28.5g	4.4g	147.7mg	4.0mg
22.1g	30.0g	24.2g	11.8g	113.5mg	4.1mg
42.1g	41.6g	54.9g	5.0g	346.7mg	3.8mg
37.4g	29.7g	23.9g	7.6g	518.5mg	7.7mg
28.9g	71.7g	17.0g	7.6g	123.8mg	2.4mg
38.3g	39.2g	23.6g	9.1g	74.1mg	4.2mg
33.4g	28.4g	42.8g	11.4g	216.7mg	5.9mg
33.7g	36.7g	25.2g	12.5g	143.2mg	7.0mg
31.2g	33.9g	41.5g	14.0g	138.8mg	7.7mg
42.7g	27.5g	49.5g	8.1g	125.9mg	7.0mg
41.6g	27.9g	63.4g	3.7g	525.2mg	3.2mg
32.0g	27.9g	35.2g	4.6g	252.0mg	4.9mg

Recipe Name	Energy	Energy
Chicken and corn soup with herb butter	876kJ	209 cal
Chicken drumstick satay, coconut rice with soy bean puree	3566kJ	852 cal
Cumberland sausage with bubble and squeak and onion sauce	3055kJ	730 cal
Italian seafood and bean stew	2462kJ	588 cal
Meatloaf with mushroom sauce and parsnip puree	2491kJ	595 cal
Salmon fillet, pease pudding and parsley sauce	3755kJ	897 cal
Semolina pizza with ricotta and basil	3554kJ	849 cal
Shepherd's pie	2171kJ	519 cal
Smoked cod brandade	3002kJ	717 cal
Bacon dust	214kJ	51 cal
Guacamole	629kJ	150 cal
Honey soy sauce	252kJ	60 cal
Lemon curd	1876kJ	448 cal
Macerated strawberries	301kJ	72 cal
Mushroom dust	151kJ	36 cal
Mushroom sauce	800kJ	191 cal
Onion Sauce	209kJ	50 cal
Parsley sauce	1350kJ	323 cal
Poached chicken breasts	443kJ	106 cal
Poached pears	1411kJ	337 cal
Quick gravy	428kJ	102 cal
Satay sauce	1074kJ	257 cal
Seedless berry compote	231kJ	55 cal

Protein	Total fat	Carbo-hydrate	Dietary fibre	Calcium	Iron
8.7g	13.8g	12.3g	2.1g	34.2mg	0.9mg
46.3g	64.2g	21.1g	6.1g	144.5mg	2.7mg
20.3g	61.9g	20.0g	9.2g	273.7mg	6.4mg
43.2g	34.0g	24.6g	9.5g	296.2mg	3.5mg
27.6g	41.0g	25.0g	10.8g	0.0mg	0.0mg
44.1g	63.1g	37.4g	7.8g	125.5mg	4.1mg
33.6	52.9g	59.7g	3.5g	785.1mg	1.5mg
35.8	27.1g	28.8g	7.9g	214.1mg	4.1mg
33.6	48.4g	35.1g	5.3g	110.6mg	2.1mg
7.7g	1.8g	0.7g	0.4g	9.5mg	0.6mg
1.7g	15.0g	1.4g	2.2g	17.3mg	0.6mg
0.7g	0.0g	14.6g	0.2g	4.4mg	0.3mg
5.1g	25.5g	52.7g	0.7g	36.3mg	0.9mg
1.8g	0.1g	15.5g	1.4g	15.0mg	0.6mg
4.8g	0.4g	2.1g	2.3g	4.3mg	0.4mg
1.8g	19.3g	3.1g	0.5g	25.8mg	0.2mg
1.6g	2.7g	4.3g	0.8g	18.3mg	0.5mg
2.4g	32.8g	5.6g	0.4g	53.6mg	0.3mg
22.3g	1.6g	0.2g	0.0g	15.1mg	0.4mg
0.3g	0.1g	85.8g	3.1g	10.9mg	0.3mg
1.6g	8.1g	5.8g	0.3g	16.0mg	0.5mg
7.9g	22.2g	5.5g	3.2g	25.7mg	1.3mg
0.6g	0.1g	12.2g	1.9g	9.7mg	0.2mg

Recipe Name	Energy	Energy
Tartare sauce	517kJ	123 cal
Tomato chutney	107kj	26 cal
Tomato sauce	244kj	58 cal
Bubble and squeak	462kj	110 cal
Carrot and orange puree	376kj	90 cal
Chick pea puree	982kj	235 cal
Coconut rice	468kj	112 cal
Creamed potato	678kj	162 cal
Creamed semolina	530kj	127 cal
Cannellini bean puree	636kj	152 cal
Easy corn puree	544kj	130 cal
Easy pea puree	471kj	112 cal
Mango puree (moulded)	249kj	60 cal
Parsnip puree	478kj	114 cal
Pea and mint puree	693kj	166 cal
Pear puree (moulded)	241kj	58 cal
Pease pudding	1102kj	263 cal
Puree pea moulds	211kj	50 cal
Refried beans	481kj	115 cal
Soy bean puree	646kj	154 cal
Spinach puree	496kj	119 cal

The figures above are estimations and the final nutrient value of the food will depend on serving size. Where a range of serves for a recipe is listed, we have used the higher number of serves. Some of the recipes recommend a food to serve with.

Protein	Total fat	Carbo-hydrate	Dietary fibre	Calcium	Iron
0.4g	10.1g	7.9g	0.2g	9.3mg	0.2mg
0.8g	0.1g	4.5g	1.1g	16.0mg	0.3mg
1.6g	3.2g	4.6g	2.1g	20.3mg	0.6mg
3.2g	4.8g	11.8g	3.4g	45.4mg	1.4mg
1.4g	5.3g	7.5g	3.5g	26.2mg	0.4mg
4.4g	18.6g	11.4g	3.3g	38.9mg	1.6mg
1.6g	5.3g	14.4g	0.4g	8.0mg	0.3mg
2.4g	12.4g	9.6g	1.5g	18.3mg	0.2mg
2.5g	6.6g	14.2g	0.6g	16.0mg	0.3mg
4.5g	9.8g	9.6g	6.3g	72.7mg	3.0mg
2.6g	6.3g	14.7g	2.5g	7.1mg	0.6mg
4.8g	5.9g	7.5g	6.2g	28.8mg	1.6mg
0.8g	0.6g	11.3g	2.5g	0.0mg	0.0mg
1.5g	7.9g	8.2g	2.2g	22.2mg	0.3mg
6.1g	10.8g	8.6g	5.8g	33.7mg	1.8mg
0.3g	0.0g	13.0g	3.0g	0.0mg	0.0mg
15.2g	6.4g	33.6g	7.5g	35.6mg	2.6mg
0.3g	0.0g	11.8g	1.8g	5.3mg	0.2mg
4.8g	5.4g	10.1g	4.7g	40.2mg	2.1mg
6.9g	12.5g	1.9g	4.6g	38.4mg	1.3mg
3.0g	9.5g	4.9g	1.2g	68.3mg	1.9mg

These have only been included in the analysis if they are listed in the ingredients. Each recipe was analysed using Foodworks 7 (Xyris, Brisbane) based on Australian food composition data.

Conversions

Our conversion charts are particularly detailed in consideration of the safety aspects of preparing texture-modified diets.

1 teaspoon = 5ml
1 tablespoon (Australian) = 4 teaspoons
1 tablespoon (UK) = 3 teaspoons (½ fl oz)
1 cup = 250 ml (8 fl oz)

1.25L	5 cups	44fl oz
1.5L	6 cups	52fl oz
2L	8 cups	70fl oz
2.5L	10 cups	88fl oz

Weight conversions

Liquid conversions

metric	cup	Imperial
60ml	¼ cup	2fl oz
100ml		3½fl oz
125ml	½ cup	4fl oz
150ml		5fl oz
185ml	¾ cup	6fl oz
200ml		7fl oz
250ml	1 cup	8¾fl oz
310ml	1¼ cups	10½fl oz
375ml	1½ cups	13fl oz
430ml	1¾ cups	15fl oz
475ml		16fl oz
500ml	2 cups	16fl oz
625ml	2½ cups	21½fl oz
750ml	3 cups	24fl oz
1L	4 cups	32fl oz

10g		¼oz	
15g		½oz	
30g		1oz	
60g		2oz	
90g		3oz	
125g		4oz	(¼lb)
155g		5oz	
185g		6oz	
220g		7oz	
250g		8oz	(½lb)
280g		9oz	
315g		10oz	
345g		11oz	
375g		12oz	(¾lb)
410g		13oz	
440g		14oz	
470g		15oz	
500g (½kg)	16oz	(1lb)	
750g		24oz	(1½lb)
1kg		32oz	(2lb)
1.5kg		48oz	(3lb)
2kg		64oz	(4lb)

Cup measures

1 cup almonds whole	110g	3½oz
1 cup flaked almonds	125g	4oz
1 cup banana mashed	240g	7½oz
1 cup basil leaves 50g		1¾oz
1 cup berries frozen	125g	4oz
1 cup breadcrumbs soft	60g	2¼oz
1 cup breadcrumbs dried	125g	4½oz
1 cup grated cheese 125g	4½oz	
1 cup couscous	190g	6¾oz
1 cup chocolate, chopped	150g	5oz
1 cup desiccated coconut 90g	3¼oz	
1 cup thickened cream	250g	8oz
1 cup plain flour	135g	4½ oz
1 cup golden syrup	380g	13oz
1 cup honey	400g	14oz
1 cup icing sugar	125g	4oz
1 cup lentils	185g	
1 cup rice	155g	5½oz
1 cup rolled oats uncooked100g	3½oz	
1 cup yoghurt 250g	8oz	
1 cup caster sugar	225g	
1 cup brown sugar	200g	

Oven temperatures

Celsius (electric)	Celsius (fan forced)	Fahrenheit	Gas mark
120°	100°	250°	1 very slow
150°	130°	300°	2 slow
180°	160°	350°	4 mod
190°	170°	375°	5 mod hot
200°	180°	400°	6 hot
230°	210°	450°	7 very hot
250°	230°	500°	9 very hot

Authors and acknowledgements

Peter Morgan-Jones

Peter has cooked for the British Royal Family and alongside some of Australia's best-known chefs and is now HammondCare's Executive Chef and Food Ambassador. Peter began work with HammondCare in 2012, after five years as Head Chef at the Art Gallery of NSW. Other culinary highlights for Peter include working in top restaurants in Bermuda, Germany and London as well as some of Sydney's most iconic restaurants including Gay Bilson's Bennelong at the Opera House, the three-hat MG Garage with Janni Kyritsis and his own one-hat Clock Hotel Restaurant.

Now Peter has embraced the opportunity to bring to the aged care sector his vast restaurant experience along with his love of 'unadulterated' food where 'the flavours do the talking' through fresh, seasonal and sustainable produce and innovation in modified meals.

Danielle McIntosh

Danielle is a Senior Dementia Consultant with The Dementia Centre, HammondCare, which offers impartial research and advice based on international best practice. Danielle is an Occupational Therapist and has considerable experience working with adults with cognitive and neurological disorders. For the past nine years Danielle has been involved in caring for people with dementia at home and in residential care, dementia-suitable design, and behavioural needs support and care planning. Danielle has been a presenter at dementia conferences nationally and internationally. She has co-authored two books on dementia care and using assistive technology in the home.

Emily Colombage

Emily is an Accredited Practising Dietitian working in residential aged care at HammondCare. Her major interests are dementia and nutrition, menu design and support and education of staff and carers. Emily was involved in the Going to Stay at Home project, speaking to carers of people living with dementia at home, about food and nutrition. She is committed to improving the lives of people living with dementia through food and raising awareness about malnutrition in the ageing population.

Prudence Ellis

Prudence is a Certified Practising Speech Pathologist and works full-time with adults with acquired speech, language and swallowing disorders. She works at HammondCare's Braeside Hospital and privately with people living in aged care homes and the community. Her areas of expertise are rehabilitation, aged care, palliative care, with a special interest in people with dementia. Prudence is passionate about improving the quality of life for people with dementia and swallowing difficulties.

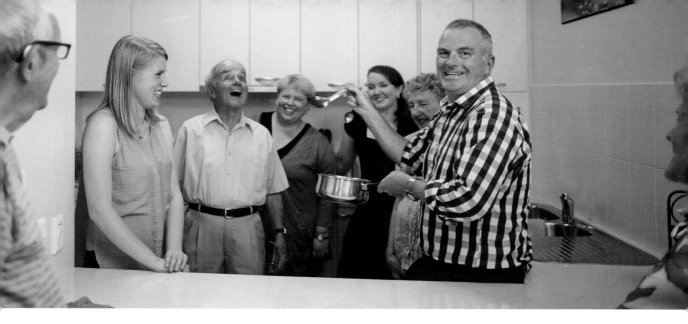

Don't give me eggs that bounce authors Emily Colombage, Danielle McIntosh, Prudence Ellis and Peter Morgan-Jones sharing a laugh and the joy of food with HammondGrove residents Keith, Rona, Ron and Jan.

Acknowledgments

The authors would like to thank the following people who through their support and contribution made this book possible: The residents, clients, families and dedicated staff from HammondCare services who provided suggestions, feedback and encouragement. The participants and staff from the Going to Stay at Home program, funded by the Australian Government Department of Social Services, who generously provided advice and feedback. Shirley Seah Szu Ying and Hui Kee Chiam who assisted with nutritional facts and research. Annalissa Roy, who as a Project Officer with the Dementia Centre, provided support with recipe reviewing. Maggie Beer, for her guidance and inspiration to make food better. Janni Kyritsis, for his advice, encouragement and being a great mentor. Also, our thanks to family, friends and colleagues who reviewed the manuscript and provided feedback and suggestions: Rebecca Morgan-Jones, Cristabel Morgan-Jones, Philippa Cahill, Jess Bottom, Carolyn Bunney, Vicky Weng, Queeny Lau, Sarah Brown, Peter Welfare, Prashanth Colombage, Kerry Gilsenan, My Phuong Ngo, Lisa Forbes, members of Speech Pathology Email ChatS (SPECS) and Rebecca Forbes.

Thanks also to HammondCare for saying no to eggs that bounce and for encouraging a rich food culture in health and aged care as part of it mission to improve quality of life for people in need.

And to the many carers and other unsung heroes of passionate food delivery in homes and services across the world, cooking tasty, nutritious and glorious food for people you love and support—bon appétit!

Index

Published by HammondCare Media (formerly HammondPress)
Sydney Australia
phallett@hammond.com.au
hammondcare.com.au dementiacentre.com.au
First published by HammondCare Media 2014

10 9 8 7 6 5 4 3 2 1

Cover and internal design: sd creative
Photography: Matt Jewell

National Library of Australia Cataloguing-in-Publications Data
Author: Morgan-Jones, Peter.
Title: Don't give me eggs that bounce: 118 cracking recipes for people with Alzheimer's / Peter Morgan-Jones, Emily Colombage, Danielle McIntosh, Prudence Ellis.
ISBN: 9780987189295 (paperback)
Notes: Includes bibliographical references and index.
Subjects: Cooking—Cooking for the sick. Alzheimer's disease—Diet therapy—Recipes.
Dewey Number: 641.563

For the latest news on *Don't give me eggs that bounce* and to share tips, recipes and feedback, visit crackingrecipes.com